PALEO COOKBOOK

QUICK AND EASY RECIPES TO LOSE WEIGHT AND GET INTO SHAPE

FRANCESCA BONHEUR

APEX UNIVERSAL LTD PTY

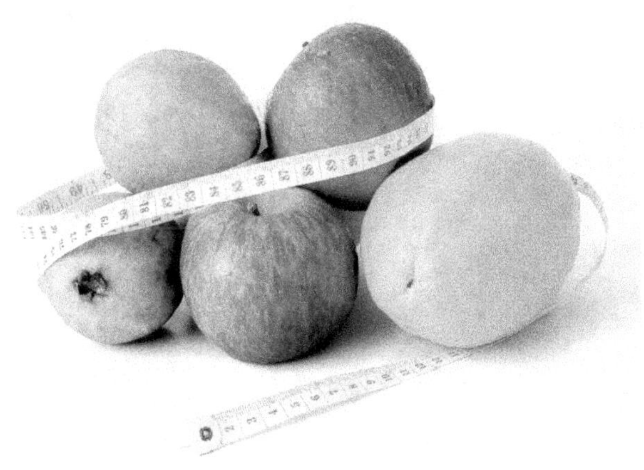

DEDICATION AND GRATITUDE

It is believed that when we express gratitude, we shall keep in mind that one of the most precious appreciation is not to thank people with simple words; but to follow those words and to practice it into reality. And we are happy to encourage you to lose weight with the help of this Paleo diet book. This book is a follow up to our first Paleo diet book and the first release of our new exciting Paleo recipe book, so please feel free to join us. This book is dedicated to you with full love and care with each recipe.

CONTENTS

ABOUT THIS BOOK

As the Paleo diet represents a very simple form of diet; we can say that it is the Natural diet that we were destined to eat and follow in the first place. Therefore, we are offering you this Paleo book which is the second in a six part series. The Paleo diet is also known as the Stone Age diet or the Primal diet. In general, a Paleo diet focuses on eating meals that are based on low carbohydrates, it is high in protein and it doesn't contain any processed or packaged foods. This Paleo book will help you learn how to adopt a new eating lifestyle diet that you will benefit from it throughout your entire life. With this Pale diet book, you can enjoy natural and delicious recipes at the same time in order to remain healthy, to lose weight and to increase the level of your energy. Whether you suffer from diabetes, heart disease, osteoporosis or even any other illness, you can start enjoying our recipes wholeheartedly to lose weight and in order to increase the level of your energy. This book will be your comprehensive and guiding book to embrace this new Paleo Lifestyle diet. And not only this Paleo book will help you remain healthy, but it will also teach you how to organize your food daily and how to eat the way we were supposed to eat since the day we were born. In this book, you will find a wide range of recipes that you will enjoy for sure. It is an original recipe book with the simplicity of its ingredients and its diversity of flavors. Stop following different diets and start your journey to a better life and good health with this Paleo Diet cook book.

CHAPTER 1

INTRODUCTION

TRYING to lose weight can be very hard sometimes, so we are offering you this Paleo book which is the second in a six part series and we want to thank you and congratulate you for downloading the book, ***"Paleo Cookbook Quick and easy Recipes to lose weight and get into shape "***.

When you think that you have lost weight, you would probably find that you have gained some extra pounds. And this makes us wonder about the main reason that makes losing weight very difficult. And while you may be wondering why losing weight has become very difficult for many of you, you may not realize that the solution is very close. It is a solution that will help you start a diet without worrying about counting the calories within your meals? Probably, you have never done that and whenever you start the process of counting calories; you won't be able to enjoy the taste of your favorite meals anymore. But what if you succeed in finding the most suitable diet for you that will let you enjoy the most delicious meals you are used to without any restrictions? Paleo diet is the best diet with which you can control your weight without depriving your body of any of your favorite dishes. Get ready to have your own doctor at home, your Self doctor Paleo diet that you will love for its health benefits, its simplicity, and because of its important role in losing weight. Experts have agreed upon this diet and have admitted its efficacy as one of the most important evolutionary diets around the globe. Paleo diet has proven that it is one of the best forms of diets since it was created. Yet, despite its importance and its efficacy, the use of a Paleo Diet was restricted as people were not attracted to the idea of using natural foods like fruits, vegetables and lean proteins. But with the rising problem of obesity and because people started looking for a healthy diet that helps lose weight in a short time; Paleo Diet found its place as the most effective diet to lose weight in a short period of time. This Paleo recipe book is a continuation of our first Paleo book and it will help you remain healthy and boost your energy as it is based on the consumption of simple and Natural ingredients. Get ready to enjoy the healthiest Paleo Diet recipes and start giving up on the unhealthy choices of food. With this Paleo book, you will be able to control your weight by mastering your appetite. And if you want to learn the secret of the Paleo Diet and its role in losing weight, then you should read our "Paleo Diet book for beginners". You will find all the information you need about losing weight in less than a month and what is more interesting about the Paleo diet books that following a Paleo diet is much more satiating than any other form of diet. With our Paleo recipes, you will eat fewer calories without having to fight the feeling of hunger. You will be able to enjoy a long and healthy life while you can still enjoy your scrumptious dishes with your family and friends. Our Paleo recipes will be mainly based on vegetables and fruits that are packed with, phytonutrients, antioxidants, minerals and vitamins. Following these Paleo diet recipes will protect you from a variety of diseases and will decrease the risk of neurological decline and the danger of diabetes.

You will notice that our recipes will be based on a wide range of food like chicken, beef, and fish and on vegetables with a dessert made of fruits. What is most special about our recipes is that our recipes will be affordable for you. And as we realize that time is a key in making any recipe, we have made sure that all our recipes are characterised by the ease of its preparation and its easy cooking directions. So don't hesitate anymore and let us get started...

CHAPTER 2
BREAKFAST PALEO RECIPES

BAKED EGGS WITH AVOCADO

- ***Cooking Time: 20 minutes***
- ***Preparation Time: 10 minutes***
- ***Servings: 2-3***

- **NOTE:**

WITH A BREAKFAST RICH IN PROTEINS, there is nothing that can be more energizing and helping you feel full for the entire day. Besides, the use of avocados makes great sources of vitamin E. Making this recipe is very simple and easy; you are going to enjoy it very much.

INGREDIENTS

- 1 Halved avocado with the stone removed
- 2 Large eggs
- 1 Pinch of salt
- 1 Pinch of ground black pepper
- ¼ Cup of crumbled cooked bacon
- ¼ Cup of fresh salsa and jalapeños.

Directions:

1. Start by preheating your oven to about 425º F
2. Halve the avocado; then remove the stone.
3. Gently, widen the pit of the avocado to allow a larger room for the egg to be scooped inside
4. Put the avocado halves into separate ramekins in a medium baking tray
5. Crack in a large egg in each of the avocado halves, then season it with a little bit of salt and with 1 pinch of pepper
6. Bake your eggs in the avocado halves in the preheated oven until the egg becomes perfectly cooked for about 15 minutes
7. Serve and enjoy!

Nutritional information

- Calories per serving – 271.3 calories
- Fat per serving – 20.2 grams
- Saturated Fats – 4.9 gram
- Total Carbs per serving –2.1 grams
- Protein per serving – 14.4 grams

SAUSAGE BALLS

- *Cooking Time: 40 minutes*
- *Preparation Time: 15 minutes*
- *Servings: 15*

- **NOTE:**

These sausage balls are great to serve at breakfast; it is delicious and nutritious at the same time. Besides, this recipe is very easy to make and you don't need more than very simple ingredients to make these delicious sausage balls.

INGREDIENTS

- 8 Slices of cut bacon
- 1 and ½ pounds of ground breakfast sausage
- ½ Diced onion
- 10 Diced Mushrooms, diced
- 1 Shredded large parsnip
- 8 Finely cut sage leaves

Directions:

1. Cook your diced bacon pieces over a medium heat for a few minutes or until the bacon becomes crispy
2. Remove the bacon from the heat and put it into a serving platter over a paper towel and set it aside to cool for a couple of minutes
3. Put the sausage into a medium mixing bowl and set it aside.
4. Add in the onion, the mushrooms and the parsnip to your food processor.
5. Slice the onion and the mushrooms; then grate your parsnip
6. Add the onion, the mushrooms and the grated parsnips to your mixing bowl; then add in the bacon pieces and the sage.
7. Preheat the oven to about 375° F and prepare a baking sheet by lining it with a parchment paper
8. Combine your ingredients altogether in a mixing bowl; then form your mixture into the size of balls
9. Arrange the obtained balls over the baking sheet and bake it in the oven for about 40 minutes
10. Remove the sausage balls from the oven and set it aside to cool for 5 minutes; then serve and enjoy it!

Nutritional information

- Calories per serving – 200.1 calories
- Fat per serving – 16.9 grams
- Saturated Fats – 2.3 gram
- Total Carbs per serving –5.1 grams
- Protein per serving – 8.3 grams

BREAKFAST TACOS

- ***Cooking Time: 10 minutes***
- ***Preparation Time: 5 minutes***
- ***Servings: 3***

- **NOTE:**

These Paleo Tortillas are very simple and easy to make that you will love it and you can even share it with your friends. It is very delicious and nutritious as well with the eggs, rich in proteins.

INGREDIENTS

- 6 Large eggs
- 1 Finely chopped green Onion stalk
- 1 Chopped Tomato
- 1 Pitted, peeled and chopped Avocado
- 4 Tablespoon of Fresh Cilantro
- 4 Tablespoons of Salsa
- 4 Tablespoons of Mexican shredded cheese
- The Juice of 1 Lime

- 1 Pinch of sea salt
- 1 Pinch of fresh ground Pepper
- Cooking spray
- 3 Paleo Wraps

Directions

1. Grease a large non - stick frying pan with cooking spray
2. Heat up a saucepan over a medium heat
3. Into a large bowl, crack in the eggs and mix it altogether with the salt, the pepper and the white part of the green onion
4. Add the mixture of the eggs to the pan; then cook it over a medium heat
5. Stir very well until your eggs are perfectly scrambled; then cook the mixture for about 4 minutes
6. Add the cooked eggs to each of your Paleo wraps
7. Top the wraps with the green onion, the tomato, the avocado, the cilantro, the salsa, the cheese, and the lime
8. Roll up your wraps like tacos and enjoy your delicious breakfast!

Nutritional information

- Calories per serving – 373 calories
- Fat per serving – 20.6 grams
- Saturated Fat – 5.3 gram
- Total Carbs per serving – 31.6 grams
- Protein per serving – 16.6 grams

BANANA PANCAKES

- ***Cooking Time: 8 minutes***
- ***Preparation Time: 5 minutes***
- ***Servings: 4***

- **NOTE:**

Have you deprived yourself of the pleasure of eating pancakes because you have chosen to follow a certain diet? What if you can enjoy a very delicious and sweet breakfast right now? If yes, then this recipe is the best choice for you; it is scrumptious by nature; you are going to love it.

INGREDIENTS

- 2 Ripe bananas
- 2 Tablespoons of chunky almond butter
- 4 Large eggs
- Chocolate chips; Dark

Directions

1. Mash the bananas into a large mixing bowl.
2. Mix the bananas with about 2 scoops of the almond butter and combine it with the eggs into your bowl
3. Whisk your ingredients very well; then prepare a flat saucepan by putting it over a medium heat
4. Scoop about ¼ cup of your mixture into the flat saucepan and wait until the bubbles start to show up
5. Flip the pancakes; then cook it for about 1 to 2 minutes
6. Top each of your pancakes with a little bit of dark chocolate chips
7. Once you have finished with the mixture and you cooked all the pancakes, serve and enjoy it
8. You can add topping fruits of your choice

Nutritional information

- Calories per serving – 275 calories
- Fat per serving – 18.2 grams
- Saturated Fat – 3.7 gram
- Total Carbs per serving –20.6 grams
- Protein per serving – 5 grams

SAUSAGE CASSEROLE

- ***Cooking Time: 35 minutes***
- ***Preparation Time: 10 minutes***
- ***Servings: 5-6***

- **NOTE:**

With this Paleo breakfast, you won't feel hungry at all. This recipe is packed with nutrients, herbs and proteins. The taste of sweet potatoes adds a unique twisting taste to your breakfast. Sausage casserole is very easy to make and also doesn't need many ingredients.

INGREDIENTS:

- ½ Pound of breakfast sausage
- 2 Cups of chopped sweet potatoes
- 3 Cups of chopped baby spinach
- 3 Cups of egg beaters
- 1 Pinch of salt
- 1 Pinch of pepper
- 2 Tablespoons of chopped pickled jalapenos

- 2 Ounces of shredded cheddar cheese
- 4 Medium, thinly sliced baby peppers

Directions:

1. Cook the sausage in a non-stick skillet over a medium heat until it is no longer pink, for about 2 minutes
2. Now, microwave the chopped sweet potato for about 4 minutes.
3. Drained any excess of fat; then add in the sweet potatoes and cook for about 2 minutes
4. Grease a baking tray with cooking spray; then combine all of your ingredients together in the baking tray and top it with a little bit of cheese
5. Top with the sliced pepper; then bake your breakfast tray in the oven for about 35minutes
6. Once the time is up; remove the tray from the oven; then set it aside to cool for about 5 minutes
7. Serve and enjoy your breakfast!

Nutritional information

- Calories per serving – 294 calories
- Fat per serving – 14.9 grams
- Saturated Fat – 2.9 gram
- Total Carbs per serving – 17 grams
- Protein per serving – 21 grams

CRANBERRY GRANOLA BARS

- ***Cooking Time: 30 minutes***
- ***Preparation Time: 5 minutes***
- ***Servings: 10***

- **NOTE:**

Whether you are resting at home or you are going for a trip; you can make this granola recipe in a very short time. These Chewy granola bars make a perfect breakfast to enjoy it with your family or even by yourself.

INGREDIENTS

- 3 Cups of whole almonds, sunflower seeds and walnuts
- 1 Cup of dried cranberries
- 2 Cups of unsweetened shredded coconut
- ¼ Cup of coconut oil
- ½ Cup of sunflower seed butter
- ½ Cup of raw honey
- ¼ Teaspoon of pure vanilla extract

- ½ Teaspoon of sea salt
- 1 Teaspoon of cinnamon

Directions

1. Prepare a baking tray by lining it with a parchment paper; then set it aside
2. Pour the nuts into a deep and large mixing bowl; then combine very well
3. Take about 1 cup of the assorted nuts out of the bowl; then put it over a cutting board. With a sharp knife; chop the nuts into small pieces
4. Take the remaining cups of the nuts; then add it to the food processor
5. Pulse your ingredients for a few seconds
6. Remove the nuts from your food processor; then put it over the cutting board and stir very well
7. Add the cranberries to your mixture; then stir very well to combine your ingredients
8. Into a deep and small pan, add the coconut oil, the sunflower seed butter, the honey, the vanilla, the salt and the cinnamon.
9. Cook your ingredients and keep stirring over a medium heat or until your ingredients start bubbling
10. Remove the ingredients from the heat; then pour the mixture over the nuts
11. Pour the mixture of the honey and the nuts into your already prepared tray that is lined with parchment paper
12. Wet your hands and firmly press your ingredients until you make sure everything is firmly packed
13. Set your mixture aside for about 2 hours
14. Cover your mixture; then put it into the freezer for about 1 hour

15. With a parchment paper; remove the granola out of the tray and place it over a cutting board
16. With a sharp knife; slice the granola to your taste
17. Serve and enjoy your granola bars!

Nutritional information

- Calories per serving – 123.2 calories
- Fat per serving – 8.7 grams
- Saturated Fat – 4.9 gram
- Total Carbs per serving – 10.5 grams
- Protein per serving – 2 grams

SCOTCH EGGS WITH GROUND MEAT

- ***Cooking Time: 35 minutes***
- ***Preparation Time: 10 minutes***
- ***Servings: 6***

- **NOTE:**

The history of scotch eggs dates back to the year of 1738 when it was first made in London. And this recipe made of scotch eggs makes one of the best breakfast recipes you can eat. It is rich in proteins and helps energize you.

INGREDIENTS:

- 6 Large eggs
- 1 Pound of ground breakfast sausage
- 2 Teaspoons of spice or herb like curry powder, sage, rosemary, mustard and parsley
- ½ Teaspoon of salt to taste

Directions:

1. Start by boiling the eggs for about 4 minutes in a saucepan; then drain the saucepan of the hot water and cover your eggs into cold water; then set it aside to cool
2. Now, peel the eggs and pat it dry with the help of paper towel.
3. Combine the ground mince with the spices and herbs of your choice
4. Take a handful of ground meat; then flatten it with your hand
5. Put the egg into the ground meat and carefully spread the mince around your egg; make sure to cover the entire egg with the minced meat
6. Put the scotch eggs in a greased baking tray and bake it into the oven for about 30 minutes at a heat of about 350° F
7. Serve and enjoy your scotch eggs!

Nutritional information

- Calories per serving – 169.1 calories
- Fat per serving – 8.3 grams
- Saturated Fat – 2.9 gram
- Total Carbs per serving –0.70 grams
- Protein per serving – 23.2 grams

SWEET POTATO FRITTERS

- ***Cooking Time: 20 minutes***
- ***Preparation Time: 5 minutes***
- ***Servings: 8***

- **NOTE:**

Who doesn't like the soothing taste of the crispy and sweet potatoes? It is a very delicious and its crispy taste will energize you for the rest of the day. Once you taste these delicious fritters, you won't be able to resist it and you will get addicted to it day by day.

INGREDIENTS

- 6 Cut bacon strips into pieces
- 2 Medium, peeled and skinned sweet potatoes
- 3 Chopped scallions
- 2 Beaten eggs
- 3 Tablespoons of coconut flour
- 1 Teaspoon of paprika

- 1 Pinch of salt
- 1 Pinch of black ground pepper

Directions

1. Start by frying the bacon pieces; then stir very well to cook it.
2. Remove the bacon from the frying pan and set it aside on paper towels to let it drain
3. Now, peel the sweet potatoes and grate it into a medium bowl
4. Add the fried bacon pieces to the potatoes
5. Add the chopped scallion; then add the whisked eggs and add about 3 tablespoons of coconut flour
6. Season with a little bit of salt and with 1 pinch of pepper; then mix very well
7. To form your fritters, scoop your mixture with about ¼ cup of a measuring cup for each of the fritters
8. Arrange the fritters over a baking tray lined with parchment paper
9. Gently flatten the fritters
10. Pour ¼ cup of oil into a skillet and heat the skillet over a medium heat
11. Cook your fritters in the non-stick skillet for about 2 to 3 minutes per each side or until your potatoes are perfectly cooked
12. Remove the fritters from the heat and let it drain over a paper towel
13. Serve and enjoy your fritters!

Nutritional information

- Calories per serving – 112.6 calories

- Fat per serving – 5.2 grams
- Saturated Fat – 3.8 gram
- Total Carbs per serving – 14.4 grams
- Protein per serving – 2.3 grams

BREAKFAST WAFFLES

- ***Cooking Time: 15 minutes***
- ***Preparation Time: 10 minutes***
- ***Servings: 5-6***

- **NOTE:**

Make your breakfast easy and light with very simple ingredients and with a very few ingredients. It is a gluten-free recipe that any of you can enjoy and it is also rich in proteins and in vitamins.

INGREDIENTS

- 2 Medium cooked and mashed sweet potatoes
- ½ Cup of almond butter
- 1 Tablespoon of coconut flour
- 3 Large eggs (Separate the yolks and the whites)
- 1 Teaspoon of pure vanilla extract
- 1 Teaspoon of pumpkin spice
- ½ Teaspoon of baking soda
- 2 Tablespoons of maple syrup

Directions:

1. Separate the yolks and the whites of eggs
2. Preheat the waffle maker
3. Put the egg whites into a bowl and set it aside
4. Add the egg yolks to a mixing bowl
5. Add the rest of the ingredients except for the egg whites to your large bowl
6. Blend your ingredients to at a low speed with the help of an electric mixer for 3 minutes
7. In another mixing bowl, beat your egg whites until it becomes stiff
8. Add the egg whites into your batter
9. Lightly grease the waffle maker with a little bit of coconut oil
10. Spoon the obtained batter into the moulds; then cook it until it gets a golden colour
11. Serve and enjoy your waffles with toppings of your choice and with fresh fruits!

Nutritional information

- Calories per serving – 284.8 calories
- Fat per serving – 8.1 grams
- Saturated Fat – 4.5 gram
- Total Carbs per serving –46 grams
- Protein per serving – 9.6 grams

CHORIZO FRITTATA

- ***Cooking Time: 25 minutes***
- ***Preparation Time: 5 minutes***
- ***Servings: 7***

- **NOTE:**

Do you want to enjoy a thick breakfast made of chorizo and mushrooms? It is packed with nutrients and you can eat it hot or cold. Get ready and make your favorite Paleo breakfast recipe.

INGREDIENTS

- 1 Tablespoon of olive oil
- ½ Pound of ground chorizo
- ½ Medium chopped onion
- 1 Minced garlic clove garlic
- ½ Cup of diced bell pepper
- 4 Oz of sliced mushrooms
- 1 Cup of sweet, shredded potatoes

- 7 Whisked eggs
- 1/3 Cup of coconut milk
- ½ Teaspoon of oregano
- 1 Pinch of salt
- 1 Pinch of black ground pepper
- Sliced optional garnish

Directions:

1. Preheat your oven to about 350° F.
2. In a heat- proof skillet and over a medium heat, place the chorizo; then cook it for a few minutes or until it gets brown
3. Remove the chorizo from the skillet and set it aside.
4. Add the onions and the bell pepper; then sauté the ingredients for about 3 minutes Add the mushrooms; then season with 1 pinch of salt and 1 Pinch of pepper
5. Cook your ingredients; then add the minced garlic and stir very well
6. Add your cooked chorizo; then add the raw and shredded sweet potato and stir very well
7. In a separate bowl, whisk altogether the coconut milk with the oregano, and 1 pinch of salt and 1 pinch of pepper.
8. Pour the egg mixture into the skillet and stir very well
9. Put the skillet in the oven and bake it at a temperature of about 350° F for about 20 minutes
10. Remove the skillet from the oven; then slice it and serve with toppings of your choice like avocado!

Nutritional information

- Calories per serving – 230 calories

- Fat per serving – 4 grams
- Saturated Fat – 4.5 gram
- Total Carbs per serving – 16.9 grams
- Protein per serving – 20.9 grams

CHAPTER 3

LUNCH RECIPES

CHICKEN SOUP

- ***Cooking Time: 40 minutes***
- ***Preparation Time: 10 minutes***
- ***Servings: 4***

- **NOTE:**

WHAT IS BETTER to start your lunch with a healthy soup; you don't need any sophisticated ingredients; all you need is a few ingredients and the taste will be unforgettable. This recipe is perfect for most the types of diets; you are going to enjoy it.

INGREDIENTS

- 2 Thinly stripped chicken breasts with the skin removed
- 1 Can of 28 oz of diced tomatoes
- 32 oz of organic chicken broth
- 1 Sweet, diced onion
- 2 Deseeded and cut jalapenos
- 3 Shredded carrots

- 2 Cups of chopped celery
- ½ to 1 bunch of chopped cilantro
- 4 Minced garlic cloves
- 1 and ½ tablespoons of tomato paste
- 1 Teaspoons of chilli powder
- 1 Teaspoon of cumin
- 1 Pinch of sea salt
- 1 Pinch of fresh ground black pepper
- 1 and ½ cups of water
- A little bit of olive oil

Directions:

1. Put a saucepan over a medium heat and add a little bit of olive oil (about 2 tablespoons)
2. Add ¼ cup of chicken broth to the saucepan and add the onions, the garlic and the jalapeno
3. Add the sea salt and the pepper; then cook until your ingredients become smooth Add the remaining chicken broth
4. Add the remaining ingredients with enough water so that you cover all the ingredients
5. Cover the soup with a lid; then let simmer over a medium heat for about 35 to 40 minutes
6. Once your chicken is perfectly cooked; remove it from the saucepan and shred it
7. Serve your soup and top it with the fresh cilantro and top it with slices of avocado

Nutritional information

- Calories per serving – 207.9 calories
- Fat per serving – 4.6 grams

- Saturated Fat – 1.3 gram
- Total Carbs per serving – 18.6 grams
- Protein per serving – 22.4 grams

- Saturated Fat – 1.3 gram
- Total Carbs per serving – 18.6 grams
- Protein per serving – 22.4 grams

BAKED CHICKEN WITH SALSA

- ***Cooking Time: 30 minutes***
- ***Preparation Time: 5 minutes***
- ***Servings: 3-4***

- **NOTE:**

If you can't decide which meal you should make, then don't hesitate anymore; you can't find any lunch better than the juicy chicken baked with salsa and served with avocado. The use of almond meal adds a crispy texture and the avocado will help you enjoy a special and flavourful lunch. Enjoy!

INGREDIENTS:

- 4 Boneless and skinless chicken breasts
- 3 Tablespoons of melted coconut oil
- 1 Cup of almond meal
- ¼ Cup of gluten-free nutritional yeast
- 1 Teaspoon of paprika
- ¼ Teaspoon of sea salt

- 1 Teaspoon of onion powder
- ½ Cup of salsa
- 1 Pitted; thinly sliced avocado

DIRECTIONS:

1. Preheat your oven to about 400° F.
2. In a medium and deep bowl, mix altogether the almond meal, the nutritional yeast, the sea salt, the paprika, and the onion powder.
3. Stir your ingredients very well and set it aside for about 1 minute
4. With a pastry brush, rub all the sides of your chicken breasts with the already melted coconut oil.
5. Put the chicken over a baking sheet or into a large baking tray; then cook your chicken for around 25 to 30 minutes
6. Remove the chicken from the oven; then set it aside to cool for about 5 minutes
7. Top the chicken with the salsa and the avocado
8. Serve and enjoy your chicken meat!

Nutritional information

- Calories per serving – 161.3 calories
- Fat per serving – 4 grams
- Saturated Fat – 0.8 gram
- Total Carbs per serving –8.2 grams
- Protein per serving – 24.7 grams

OVEN BAKED CHICKEN WITH ROSEMARY

- ***Cooking Time: 15 minutes***
- ***Preparation Time: 10 minutes***
- ***Servings: 2-3***

- **NOTE:**

This chicken recipe is easy to make and very scrumptious. You are going to like the taste of chicken; which is rich in proteins and in various zesty tastes. If you don't like chicken, you are going to change your mind for sure when you learn this recipe; it is irresistible and packed with healthy flavors.

INGREDIENTS

- 2 pounds of boneless chicken breasts
- ½ Cup of fresh-squeezed lemon juice
- 1 Tablespoon of extra virgin olive oil
- 1 Tablespoon of fresh rosemary
- 1 Minced garlic clove
- ¼ Teaspoon of sea salt

- ¼ Teaspoon of black pepper

Directions

1. In a deep and large bowl; mix altogether the olive oil, the lemon juice, the garlic, the rosemary, the salt and the pepper; then set the mixture aside.
2. Pound your chicken breasts; then cut it into thin strips
3. Put the chicken into a large bowl; then pour the marinade over it
4. Toss the chicken to coat it very well; then cover it and refrigerate it for about 2 hours
5. Preheat your grill for about 10 minutes over a medium-high heat and place the chicken over it
6. Grill your chicken meat for about 4 minutes for each side
7. Serve and enjoy your chicken!

Nutritional information

- Calories per serving – 122.1 calories
- Fat per serving – 1 grams
- Saturated Fat – 0.8 gram
- Total Carbs per serving –0.6 grams
- Protein per serving – 25.9 grams

BAKED CHICKEN WITH OLIVES

- ***Cooking Time: 40 minutes***
- ***Preparation Time: 15 minutes***
- ***Servings: 6***

- **NOTE:**

An easy to make, exotic chicken recipe, which is low in carbohydrates, this recipe is grain free and Paleo. The directions are super easy to follow and you won't need any help from any other person to make this incredibly delicious chicken lunch, you are going to enjoy it.

INGREDIENTS

- 4 Pounds of bone-in chicken thighs
- 1 Pinch black ground pepper
- 1 Pinch of salt
- 1 Jar of 16 Oz of quartered artichoke hearts
- 8 Oz of pitted, halved kalamata olives
- 9 Oz of large pimento, Spanish stuffed olives

* 10 large grated garlic cloves
* 1 Can of 15 Oz chopped tomatoes
* ½ Cup of extra virgin olive oil
* ¼ Cup of apple cider vinegar
* 2 Tablespoons of balsamic vinegar
* 1 Tablespoon of dried thyme
* 2 Tablespoons of Greek oregano

Directions

1. Rinse the chicken and pat dry it; then season it with salt and pepper.
2. Set your ingredients aside to marinade
3. In a large and deep bowl; mix all of your ingredients except for the chicken
4. Add the chicken and combine your ingredients very well; then set the chicken aside to marinate for about 3 hours or for an overnight
5. Once you are ready to cook the chicken; preheat your oven to about 450°
6. Put the chicken in a baking tray and cover it with an aluminium foil paper
7. Bake the chicken in the oven for about 40 minutes
8. Remove the chicken tray from your oven; then serve and enjoy it.

Nutritional information

* Calories per serving – 299.1 calories
* Fat per serving – 16 grams
* Saturated Fat – 3.9 gram
* Total Carbs per serving –4 grams
* Protein per serving – 29 grams

CHICKEN WITH MUSHROOM SAUCE

- ***Cooking Time: 10 minutes***
- ***Preparation Time: 5 minutes***
- ***Servings: 3-4***

- **NOTE:**

This Paleo chicken recipe is made with great care and with very nutritious ingredients. It is an extremely tasty recipe that you will enjoy with the combination of mushrooms and chicken. The addition of garlic adds a spicy taste to the dish.

INGREDIENTS

- 1 and ½ pounds of chicken thighs or skinless chicken breasts
- 1 Cup of sliced mushrooms
- ½ Tablespoon of avocado oil
- ⅛ Teaspoon of sea salt
- ⅛ Teaspoon of black pepper

- 2 Tablespoon of butter; divided
- 3 Minced garlic cloves
- ⅓ Cup of white cooking wine
- ½ Teaspoon of arrowroot powder

Directions:

1. Sprinkle the chicken with a little bit of salt and with 1 pinch of pepper.
2. In a large, non-stick skillet and over a medium high heat, sear the chicken in about ½ tablespoon of oil for about 5 minutes over each side
3. Remove the chicken from the skillet; then put it over a platter and set it aside
4. In the same skillet; melt about 1 tablespoon of butter over a medium heat; then add the minced garlic and the sliced mushrooms
5. Stir your ingredients very well; then sauté altogether until the mushrooms get a brown colour.
6. Add the wine to your pan and stir very thoroughly.
7. In a small and deep bowl mix; mix about 1 tablespoon of butter with ½ teaspoon of the arrowroot powder and smash the arrowroot powder into your butter with the help of a fork
8. Add the butter to the mixture of the mushroom and wine; then stir over a medium heat for about 6 minutes
9. Put the chicken in a serving later; then pour the mushroom sauce over the top
10. Serve and enjoy your lunch!

Nutritional information

- Calories per serving – 360.1 calories

- Fat per serving – 12 grams
- Saturated Fat – 2.6 gram
- Total Carbs per serving –4.1 grams
- Protein per serving – 49 grams

GARLIC CHICKEN WITH RED ONION

- ***Cooking Time: 20 minutes***
- ***Preparation Time: 10 minutes***
- ***Servings: 5***

- **NOTE:**

Can you think of something better than a comforting and warming garlic chicken dish that combines the taste of chicken with the taste of potatoes? Once you try it, you are going to realize how delicious this dish is and how you will get addicted to cooking it day after day!

INGREDIENTS:

- 5 to 6 skinless chicken thigh fillets
- 2 Tablespoons of olive oil
- 1 Pound of sweet potatoes
- 2 Medium red onions
- 8 Minced garlic cloves
- 2 Teaspoons of dried thyme leaves

- 1 Teaspoons of dried rosemary
- 1 Pinch of salt
- 1 Pinch of freshly ground black pepper
- 1 Teaspoon of smoked paprika
- 2 Medium lemons
- 1 Cup of chicken stock

Direction:

1. Cut each of the chicken thigh fillet in about two halves and sear it over a medium high heat in a large skillet for a few minutes
2. Cover the chicken and set it aside; meanwhile, peel your sweet potatoes and cut it into slices of about 1 and ½ cm thickness
3. Peel your vegetables and quarter your onions; then add it altogether to a saucepan with the remaining quantity of oil, the minced garlic, the herbs and the seasonings
4. Roast your vegetables at a degree of about 390° F for about 15 minutes
5. Remove the saucepan from the oven, then flip vegetable pieces with a spatula and add the chicken thighs
6. Squeeze a little bit of lemon juice over your ingredients; then adjust the seasoning with smoked paprika
7. Pour the chicken stock over the chicken and the roasted vegetables in a saucepan; then cook over a medium heat for about 20 minutes
8. Serve and enjoy your chicken and sweet potato dish with a salad or avocado slices.

Nutritional information

- Calories per serving – 298.2 calories

- Fat per serving – 18.7 grams
- Saturated Fat – 3.2 gram
- Total Carbs per serving – 16.1 grams
- Protein per serving – 20.1 grams

SPICY CHICKEN WITH CAULIFLOWER

- ***Cooking Time: 50 minutes***
- ***Preparation Time: 20 minutes***
- ***Servings: 4***

- **NOTE:**

Don't you agree that cauliflower represents one of the most delicious and versatile ingredients that you can prepare everything with it. This dish is packed with anti- inflammatory ingredients. It is a delicious dish that is packed with vitamins. You are going to enjoy your lunch with your friends and show them that you can cook like a master chef or even better.

INGREDIENTS

- 1 and ½ Pounds of Chicken Breasts
- 1 Head of Cauliflower
- 1 Teaspoon of Salt
- ½ Teaspoon of Black Pepper
- 2 Tablespoons ofOlive Oil

- 1 Large diced sweet onion
- 8 Oz of quartered Cremini Mushrooms
- 10 Oz of spinach
- 1 Canof Coconut Milk
- 1 Cup of chicken Broth
- 3 Large beaten eggs
- ½ Teaspoon of Nutmeg

INGREDIENTS

1. Remove the core of the head of cauliflower; then break it into little florets
2. Transfer the cauliflower into a food processor; then fill it with about ¾ of fullness
3. Pulse your cauliflower in the food processor and transfer it to a bowl; then repeat the same process with the remaining quantity of cauliflower until you obtain a smooth mixture
4. Squeeze your cauliflower rice with a dry and clean cloth in order to remove any excess of liquid
5. Transfer your cauliflower rice to a baking tray; then season your chicken breasts with about ½ teaspoon of the salt and about ¼ teaspoon of the black pepper.
6. In a large skillet, heat about 1 tablespoon of the olive oil over a medium-high heat.
7. Toss in the chicken and sauté it for about 6 minutes
8. Transfer your chicken to a clean cutting board and when it becomes cool; shred it into small pieces
9. Add the chicken meat to the cauliflower rice into the baking tray
10. Preheat your oven to about 325°F; meanwhile; heat about 1 tablespoon of oil in a skillet and add to it the onion with the olive oil

11. Stir in the mushrooms and sauté altogether for around 5 minutes
12. Add the spinach in and cook your ingredients until it becomes tender
13. Transfer the obtained mixture to a baking tray
14. Pour the chicken broth with the coconut milk, the eggs, the nutmeg and the remaining salt; then season with the black pepper.
15. Bake your ingredients for about 45 minutes
16. Remove the tray from the oven; then set it aside to cool for about 10 minutes
17. Serve and enjoy your dish!

Nutritional information

- Calories per serving – 241.1 calories
- Fat per serving – 9.8 grams
- Saturated Fat – 2.2 gram
- Total Carbs per serving –9.2 grams
- Protein per serving – 26.2 grams

CHICKEN, ZUCCHINI RATATOUILLE

- ***Cooking Time: 45 minutes***
- ***Preparation Time: 10 minutes***
- ***Servings: 3***

- **NOTE:**

Chicken Ratatouille is one of the most delicious dishes that you can ever taste. It is a healthy recipe that you can make with very simple ingredients and you can add your favorite herbs to it.

INGREDIENTS

- 1 Eggplant of a medium size
- 1 Medium, red bell pepper
- 2 Zucchini of a medium size
- 1 Tablespoon of Italian seasoning
- 2 Cups of tomato sauce
- 1 and ½ pounds of boneless and skinless chicken breasts
- 2 Tablespoons of olive oil
- 2 Tablespoons of fresh basil

- 1/8 Teaspoon of sea salt
- 1/8 Teaspoon of black pepper

Directions:

1. Preheat your oven to about 390° F.
2. With a sharp knife, slice your vegetables as thin as you can
3. Layer the vegetables into a casserole tray and season very well with salt and pepper
4. Season with the Italian seasoning between the layers and top with the chicken; then drizzle with the olive oil
5. Cover your dish with an aluminium foil paper; then bake your casserole in the oven for about 40 to 45 minutes
6. Remove the casserole from the oven; then top it with the basil and set it aside to cool for a few minutes
7. Serve and enjoy your nutritious chicken casserole!

Nutritional information

- Calories per serving – 103.7 calories
- Fat per serving – 1.1 grams
- Saturated Fat – 0.1 gram
- Total Carbs per serving –23.1 grams
- Protein per serving – 3.9 grams

Recipe 19: Ground chicken Peccadillo
(Cooking Time: 20 minutes\ Preparation Time: 5 minutes \ Servings: 2-3)

- **NOTE:**

This chicken recipe is perfect to serve on special occasions and what is more exciting about it is that you can also reheat it and enjoy its delicious taste. Wait no more and make your delicious recipe. You are going to enjoy this chicken peccadillo and you can also make it any time you wait even for a simple dinner.

INGREDIENTS

- 2 Tablespoons of olive oil
- 3 Medium, finely chopped garlic cloves
- 1 Medium, finely chopped yellow onion finely
- 1 Medium, finely chopped red bell pepper
- 1 and ½ pounds of Ground Chicken
- 2 Teaspoons of kosher salt
- 1 Teaspoon of black pepper
- 1 Teaspoon of paprika
- 1 Teaspoon of dried oregano
- 1 Teaspoon of ground cumin
- 1 to 2 dried bay leaves
- 1 Cup of canned, non salted chopped tomatoes
- 1 Tablespoon of tomato paste
- ¼ Cup of chopped Pimento Stuffed olives
- 2 Tablespoons of olive brine
- 2 Tablespoons of water
- 1 Tablespoon of raisins
- 1 Handful of chopped fresh cilantro

Directions:

1. Peel; then chop the garlic or finely mince it with the onion
2. Remove the cores of the olives and deseed the bell pepper
3. Mix the spices into a small tray; then slice the olives, the raisins, the tomatoes and the tomato paste; then add the olive brine and the water
4. Heat a skillet over a medium heat and once your

ingredients become hot, add the olive oil with the garlic, the onion and the bell pepper

5. Sauté your ingredients for about 7 minutes and keep stirring until your onions become translucent.
6. Add in the Ground Chicken and after that raise the heat to medium
7. With a wooden spatula; break the ground pieces of chicken with a spatula
8. Toss in the salt, the pepper, the paprika, the oregano; the cumin and the bay leaf. Cook your ingredients and stir it until it is perfectly mixed
9. Add the diced tomatoes, the tomato paste, the sliced olives, the olive juice and the water
10. Add the raisins and toss very well to mix your ingredients; then let simmer for about 20 minutes
11. Stir in the chopped cilantro; then serve over the cauliflower rice or the steamed white rice.
12. Enjoy your chicken Peccadillo!

Nutritional information

- Calories per serving – 178.4 calories
- Fat per serving – 7.7 grams
- Saturated Fat – 1 gram
- Total Carbs per serving –7.8 grams
- Protein per serving – 20.4 grams

CHICKEN, LETTUCE SALAD

- ***Cooking Time: 10 minutes***
- ***Preparation Time: 5 minutes***
- ***Servings: 5***

- **NOTE:**

This Paleo chicken salad is easy to make, rich in flavor and very healthy. Chicken salad makes a great choice for a hot summer's day; you can make your chicken salad on the go; it needs no more than a few ingredients to enjoy this zesty and flavorful salad.

INGREDIENTS

- 4 Boneless and skinless chicken breasts
- 4 Cups of chopped romaine lettuce
- 1 Chopped cucumber
- 1 Red and thinly sliced onion
- 1 Cup of halved grape tomatoes
- For the marinade:

- ¼ Cup of olive oil
- 3 Tablespoons of lemon juice
- 4 Minced garlic cloves
- 1 Teaspoon of ground cumin
- 1 Teaspoon of paprika
- ¼ Teaspoon of turmeric
- 1 Pinch of sea salt
- 1 Pinch of freshly ground black pepper
- ¾ Cup of extra virgin olive oil
- ¼ Cup of fresh lemon juice
- 2 Minced garlic cloves
- The Zest of 1 lemon;
- Fresh ground black pepper and sea salt

Directions:

1. In a small and deep bowl, combine all the ingredients of the marinade
2. Put the chicken into the marinade and refrigerate it for about 30 minutes
3. Preheat your grill to a medium high heat; then grill the chicken over the grill for about 15 minutes
4. Remove the chicken from the grill and set it aside; then combine the ingredients of the dressing
5. Slice your chicken meat into strips; then assemble your salad into a large and a big bowl and combine the romaine lettuce, the cucumber, the red onion, the tomatoes, and the lemon dressing
6. Gently toss your chicken salad
7. Serve and enjoy your chicken salad!

Nutritional information

- Calories per serving – 123.1 calories

- Fat per serving – 8.2 grams
- Saturated Fat – 2.7 gram
- Total Carbs per serving –3.2 grams
- Protein per serving – 11.1 grams

CHICKEN NUGGETS

- ***Cooking Time: 12 minutes***
- ***Preparation Time: 7 minutes***
- ***Serves: 4***

- **NOTE:**

This recipe of Crispy Chicken Nuggets makes a great choice for a quick lunch. It is an easy to make recipe and it is affordable with a few ingredients. No one can resist the taste of chicken nuggets.

INGREDIENTS

- 1 Pound of boneless and skinless chicken breasts
- ¼ Cup of almond flour
- ¾ Teaspoon of salt
- 1 Teaspoon of garlic powder
- 1 Teaspoon of paprika
- ⅛ Teaspoon of cayenne pepper
- ⅛ Teaspoon of ground black pepper
- ¼ Cup of avocado oil

Directions:

1. Cut the chicken into small pieces of about 1 and ½ inches each
2. Mix the flour with the seasonings and season the chicken with it
3. Melt the coconut oil and drizzle it over the chicken
4. Bake the seasoned chicken in a preheated oven at a degree of about 425° F for about 12 minutes
5. Once the chicken nuggets are perfectly cooked, serve and enjoy it!

Nutritional information

- Calories per serving – 250.1 calories
- Fat per serving – 18.9 grams
- Saturated Fat – 2.1 gram
- Total Carbs per serving –9 grams
- Protein per serving – 24.9 grams

CHICKEN WITH ORANGE AND PECANS

- ***Cooking Time: 12 minutes***
- ***Preparation Time: 7 minutes***
- ***Servings: 4***

- **NOTE:**

This chicken recipe is made with simple ingredients and has many nutritional benefits. The taste of the zesty juice adds a special flavor that you won't forget. Besides, the use of pecans enriches this recipe with great, healthy benefits, the most important of which is to help you lose weight.

INGREDIENTS

- 1 and ½ pounds of cubed chicken breasts
- 3 Tablespoons of coconut oil
- ½ Cup of chopped pecans
- 1 Diced yellow onion
- 1 Sliced orange bell pepper
- The juice of 1 medium orange

- The juice of 1 lemon
- 1 Cup of low sodium chicken broth
- ½ Teaspoon of salt

Directions:

1. Preheat your oven at about 350° F degrees
2. Pour about 1 to 2 tablespoons of coconut oil in a non-stick saucepan over a medium heat; then sauté the chicken on both its sides
3. Set the chicken aside in a bowl; then add about 1 tablespoon of oil and sauté the onion and the peppers for a few minutes
4. Add the broth, the juice of the orange and the lemon; then add the chicken, and let simmer for about 15 minutes; meanwhile, put the pecans in a tray covered with a parchment paper and sprinkle with a little bit of salt, chilli powder and cayenne
5. Bake the pecans for about 5 minutes in the preheated oven
6. Set the pecans aside to cool; then add it to your pan and stir very well
7. Serve and enjoy your dish!

Nutritional information

- Calories per serving – 250.1 calories
- Fat per serving – 18.9 grams
- Saturated Fat – 2.1 gram
- Total Carbs per serving –9 grams
- Protein per serving – 24.9 grams

CHICKEN FAJITAS

- *Cooking Time: 25 minutes*
- *Preparation Time: 5 minutes*
- *Servings: 3*

- **NOTE:**

This recipe of chicken fajitas makes a perfect meal to serve for special occasions. The flavorful and the colorful bell peppers add a unique twist to the chicken fajitas. It is a light and healthy recipe. The use of onion enriches the fajitas with its protective and immune power.

INGREDIENTS

- 4 Butterflied chicken breasts
- 1 Sliced bell pepper
- 1 Sliced red onion
- The juice of 1 lime
- ¼ Cup of olive oil
- 1 Minced garlic clove

- 2 Tablespoon of fresh cilantro
- ½ Teaspoon of cumin
- 1 Teaspoon of chilli powder
- 1 Teaspoon of dried oregano
- ¼ Teaspoon of cayenne pepper
- 1 Pinch of sea salt
- 1 Pinch of freshly ground black pepper
- Fresh chopped cilantro

Directions:

1. Preheat the grill to a medium-high heat.
2. In a large bowl, combine altogether the lime juice, the olive oil, the garlic, the fresh cilantro, the cumin, the chilli powder, the oregano, and the cayenne pepper
3. Season the chicken with a little bit of salt and 1 pinch of pepper to taste.
4. Put half of the mixture of the spice in a medium bowl; then add the bell pepper and the onion.
5. Arrange the chicken and fill it with the onion, the bell pepper, and the mixture of the spice.
6. Now, roll the chicken meat tightly and secure it with toothpicks
7. Brush the chicken with the mixture of the spice
8. Grill your chicken meat over a medium-high heat for about 25 minutes and flip it every 5 minutes
9. Serve and enjoy your chicken fajitas

Nutritional information

- Calories per serving – 259.1 calories

- Fat per serving – 7.9 grams
- Saturated Fat – 2.12 gram
- Total Carbs per serving – 17.5 grams
- Protein per serving – 30.7 grams

CHICKEN CURRY

- ***Cooking Time: 25 minutes***
- ***Preparation Time: 5 minutes***
- ***Servings: 4***

- **NOTE:**

Chicken curry has always been one of the favorite dishes to serve. The coconut milk makes this curry recipe creamy and flavorful. You can also add chicken stock and herbs of your choice like Garam Masala, ginger, chilies, and other spicy flavorings. You can also store your chicken curry and serve it the following day.

INGREDIENTS

- 11 Chicken drumsticks
- 1 Finely chopped onion
- 4 Minced garlic cloves
- 2 Cups of tomato sauce
- 1 Cup of chicken stock

* 1 Cup of coconut milk
* 1 Tablespoon of grated fresh ginger
* 2 Tablespoons of Garam Masala
* 2 Teaspoons of paprika
* ½ Teaspoon of ground cinnamon
* 1 Teaspoon of chilli flakes
* Fresh minced cilantro
* Coconut oil
* 1 Pinch of sea salt
* 1 Pinch of freshly ground black pepper

Directions:

1. Melt a little bit of coconut oil in a large non-stick skillet over a medium-high heat.
2. Sauté the chicken drumsticks on all of the sides; then remove the chicken and set it aside
3. Add the garlic, the onion and the ginger and sauté the ingredients until it becomes fragrant
4. Add the tomato sauce, the chicken stock and let them simmer for about 4 minutes; keep stirring from time to time
5. Return the chicken meat to the skillet; then let simmer for about 15 minutes
6. Stir in the coconut milk and adjust the seasoning with salt and pepper
7. Let the chicken curry simmer for about 5 minutes; then serve and enjoy with cilantro topping!

Nutritional information

* Calories per serving – 291 calories
* Fat per serving – 2.49 grams

- Saturated Fat – 0.7 gram
- Total Carbs per serving –30.9 grams
- Protein per serving – 37.7 grams

BAKED CHICKEN WITH GREEN BEANS

- ***Cooking Time: 60 minutes***
- ***Preparation Time: 15 minutes***
- ***Servings: 3***

- **NOTE:**

This is an affordable recipe to make chicken with; it is delicious with the rich flavors it has. The combination of tomato sauce with the green beans makes a great natural melting taste that you will like, for sure. Besides, this recipe provides is rich in proteins.

INGREDIENTS

- 6 Bone on; chicken thighs
- 1 Teaspoon of vegetable oil
- ½ Medium, chopped onion
- 1 Minced garlic clove
- 1/8 Teaspoon of turmeric
- 3 Tablespoon of tomato paste
- 2 Cups of water

- ½ Teaspoon of salt
- ½ Teaspoon of pepper
- 2 Small sweet potatoes
- 2 Cups of green beans

Directions:

1. Preheat your oven to about 400° F.
2. Arrange the chicken thighs over a square casserole dish.
3. Season your chicken generously with pepper and salt.
4. Bake your chicken uncovered for about 50 minutes.
5. Prepare the sauce: put a medium saucepan over a medium high heat and add the onions, the garlic and the turmeric; then stir very well in order to coat the onions
6. Sauté the onion for about 4 minutes
7. Add the tomato paste, the water, the salt and the pepper; then stir very well until your ingredients are combined.
8. Add the potatoes and let simmer for about 10 minutes.
9. Remove the chicken from the oven and pour the sauce on top of it
10. Place the chicken dish back in your oven; then bake it for about 20 minutes
11. Remove the chicken from the oven; then serve and enjoy it!

Nutritional information

- Calories per serving – 349 calories
- Fat per serving – 2.2 grams
- Saturated Fat – 0.6 gram
- Total Carbs per serving –33.5 grams
- Protein per serving – 43.5 grams

BAKED DUCK BREAST

- ***Cooking Time: 45 minutes***
- ***Preparation Time: 10 minutes***
- ***Servings: 4***

- **NOTE:**

With the flavorful spices, this recipe is more than tempting. The taste of the freshly ground spices in a mortar and the pestle adds a special taste to your meal. It is a meal rich in flavors and in proteins. What are you waiting for; get ready to make your delicious duck recipe.

INGREDIENTS:

- 4 Skin on duck breasts
- 14 Oz of cubed butternut squash
- 8 Thinly sliced shiitake mushrooms
- 2 Sliced small leeks
- ½ Cup of vegetable or duck stock
- 1 or 2 star anise
- ½ Teaspoon of black peppercorns

* 1 Teaspoon of sea Salt
* 2 Tablespoons of extra-virgin olive oil
* 1 Pinch of Sea salt
* 1 Pinch of freshly ground black pepper

Directions:

1. Cut the duck skin into a crisscross pattern.
2. Crush; then grind altogether the star anise, the black peppercorn, and the sea salt into a mortar; then pestle it.
3. Now, rub the ground spices over the skin of the duck skin
4. Put the duck into a container and pour in the duck stock
5. Cover the duck and set it aside to marinate for about 1 hour
6. Preheat the oven to about 350° F.
7. Put the shiitake mushrooms, the cubed butternut squash and the leeks into a roasting saucepan; then season it very well
8. Cover the saucepan and cook in the oven for about 30 minutes
9. In a large skillet and over a high heat, sear the duck meat with the skin side down
10. Put the duck breast over a rack on top of a roasting pan with the skin side up; then roast for about 15 minutes
11. Serve the duck meat with the vegetable mixture
12. Enjoy!

Nutritional information

* Calories per serving – 153 calories
* Fat per serving – 2.1 grams
* Saturated Fat – 0.0 gram
* Total Carbs per serving –8.2 grams
* Protein per serving – 25 grams

HONEY GLAZED CHICKEN BREASTS

- ***Cooking Time: 5 minutes***
- ***Preparation Time: 5 minutes***
- ***Servings: 2-3***

- **NOTE:**

This honey glazed chicken recipe is irresistible with its extra- delicious ingredients. Chicken meat is a great type of meat; the majority of the people love it and they cook it at home. You are going to learn from this recipe that chicken meat is a versatile type of meat that can be used in Paleo diet and you are going to enjoy it.

INGREDIENTS:

- 4 Skin-on duck breasts
- 1 Pinch of sea salt
- 1 Pinch of freshly ground black pepper
- 1/3 Cup of balsamic vinegar
- ¼ Cup of raw honey
- ½ Teaspoon of pure vanilla extract

- ½ Cup of chopped walnuts

Directions:

1. Combine the vinegar, the honey, and the vanilla into a small bowl.
2. Heat a heavy and large skillet over a medium heat.
3. Season the duck with a little bit of salt and 1 pinch of pepper.
4. Put the duck breasts with its skin side down, into the pan; then cook for about 10 minutes
5. Flip the duck and sauté for about 5 minutes
6. Transfer the duck to a dish and cover it with a foil; then pour the duck fat in a medium container.
7. Add the vinegar mixture and the walnuts to the large skillet and deglaze your pan
8. Stir the duck meat in the pan and flip it for several times
9. Serve your glazed duck breast immediately and enjoy this delicious taste!

Nutritional information

- Calories per serving – 194.1 calories
- Fat per serving – 1.6 grams
- Saturated Fat – 0.4 gram
- Total Carbs per serving – 17.7 grams
- Protein per serving – 26.2 grams

Recipe 28: Chicken almond flour loaf
(Cooking Time: 25 minutes \ Preparation Time: 5 minutes \ Servings: 5)

- **NOTE:**

If you desperately want to taste a delicious meatloaf and you don't have beef meat, then this recipe is the best for you. This Paleo chicken, meatloaf is rich in nutritious flavors and healthy ingredients.

INGREDIENTS

- 2 Pounds of Ground Chicken
- 2 Whisked eggs
- 1 Cup of almond flour
- 1 Cup of chopped fresh basil
- 1 Tablespoon of garlic powder
- 1 Tablespoon of onion powder
- 1 Teaspoon of dried parsley
- 1 Pinch of salt
- 1 Pinch of pepper

Directions:

1. Preheat your oven to about 375° F.
2. Mix all of your ingredients in a large bowl.
3. Put the ingredients into two medium loaf pans.
4. Bake your meat loaves for about 25 minutes in a preheated oven
5. Once the time is up, remove the chicken loaves from the oven and set it aside for about 5 minutes
6. Serve and enjoy your meat loaves
7. Eat and enjoy!

Nutritional information

- Calories per serving – 124.8 calories
- Fat per serving – 5.1 grams
- Saturated Fat – 1.3 gram
- Total Carbs per serving –8.5 grams
- Protein per serving – 11.5 grams

FRIED CHICKEN WITH APPLES

- ***Cooking Time: 20 minutes***
- ***Preparation Time: 10 minutes***
- ***Servings: 3***

- **NOTE:**

With the combination of the sweet potatoes, the apples, the Brussels sprouts and the bacon, this recipe makes a healthy Paleo chicken recipe that you will enjoy. This recipe is packed with vitamins and nutrients.

INGREDIENTS:

- 1 Tablespoon of olive oil
- 1 Pound of boneless and skinless, cubed chicken breasts
- 1 Teaspoon of kosher salt
- ½ Teaspoon of black pepper
- 4 Chopped slices of thick-cut bacon
- 3 Cups of quartered and trimmed Brussels sprouts

- 1 Medium, peeled and cubed sweet potato
- 1 Medium, chopped onion
- 2 Peeled and cored, cubed apples
- 4 Minced garlic cloves
- 2 Teaspoons of chopped fresh thyme
- 1 Teaspoon of ground cinnamon
- 1 Cup of reduced-sodium chicken broth

Directions:

1. Start by heating the oil into a non-stick skillet over a medium-high heat
2. Toss in the chicken and sprinkle a little bit of kosher salt
3. Season with a little bit of ground black pepper.
4. Cook the chicken for about 6 minutes; then transfer it to a dish lined with a paper towel
5. Lower the heat and add the bacon to the skillet and sauté it for about 7 minutes
6. Remove the bacon from the skillet and toss in the Brussels sprouts
7. Add the sweet potatoes, the onion and 1 pinch of salt
8. Cook for about 9 minutes
9. Add the garlic, the apples, the thyme, and the cinnamon; then cook for about 30 seconds
10. Add about ½ cup of broth; then let boil for about 3 minutes
11. Add the remaining quantity of chicken and add about ½ cup of broth.
12. Cook the chicken for about 2 minutes
13. Serve and enjoy!

Nutritional information

- Calories per serving – 318 calories

- Fat per serving – 10.9 grams
- Saturated Fat – 2.9 gram
- Total Carbs per serving – 25.9 grams
- Protein per serving – 31.9 grams

BAKED CHICKEN WITH SPAGHETTI SQUASH

- ***Cooking Time: 90 minutes***
- ***Preparation Time: 20 minutes***
- ***Servings: 6***

- **NOTE:**

Have you ever tried one of the delicious chicken casserole recipes? If you haven't tried it yet, it is the right time to roll up your sleeves and enjoy this healthy and scrumptious chicken dish. All the ingredients of this recipe are healthy and nutritious.

INGREDIENTS

- 2 and ½ pounds of medium spaghetti squash
- 4 Tablespoons of coconut oil
- 2 Minced garlic cloves
- 1 Diced medium carrot
- 2 Diced stalks of celery
- 1/2 Minced medium yellow onion
- 1 Small, diced red bell pepper

- 1 Pound of ground chicken
- 1 Teaspoon of garlic powder
- 1 Teaspoon of fine sea salt
- ¼ Teaspoon of black pepper
- 1 Cup of hot sauce
- 1/4 Cup of Super Simple
- 3 Large eggs, chopped and whisked chopped scallions
- 1 Sliced avocado

Directions:

1. Preheat your oven to about 390°F.
2. Cut the spaghetti squash into two halves; then place the squash on top of a baking sheet
3. Bake the squash spaghetti for about 30 minutes
4. Remove the squash from the oven; then lower the temperature to about 350°F.
5. Grease a medium baking tray with cooking spray and remove its threads
6. Set the squash aside to cool for a few minutes
7. Transfer the squash threads to a greased baking tray
8. In a large skillet and over a medium heat, melt about 2 tablespoons of coconut oil.
9. Add the carrots, the garlic, the celery, the onion, and the bell pepper; then cook for about 9 minutes
10. Add the garlic powder, the ground chicken, the salt, and the pepper; then cook for a few minutes; about 7 minutes
11. Remove the skillet from the heat and add the sauce and the mayonnaise; then stir very well
12. Pour the mixture of the chicken and add to it the spaghetti squash threads in a baking tray.
13. Add the eggs and mix very well
14. Bake the tray in the oven for about 55 minutes

15. Garnish the tray with the chopped scallion and with avocado slices.
16. Serve and enjoy!

Nutritional information

- Calories per serving – 228 calories
- Fat per serving –8.1 grams
- Saturated Fat – 3.9 gram
- Total Carbs per serving –16 grams
- Protein per serving – 13.9 grams

BEEF LUNCH RECIPES

BAKED BEEF CASSEROLE

- *Cooking Time: 40 minutes*
- *Preparation Time: 10 minutes*
- *Servings: 4*

- **NOTE:**

This baked Beef casserole is made of a variety of veggies. It is a recipe that everyone likes with the delicious and hearty taste of beef, packed with nutrients and health benefits. You are going to enjoy making this dish by yourself as it is not sophisticated. All you have to do is to follow simple directions.

INGREDIENTS

- 2 Tablespoon of olive oil
- 1 Medium; thinly sliced onion
- 2 Medium, minced garlic cloves
- 1 Tablespoon of Italian seasoning
- 1 Pound of ground beef
- 2 Medium; thinly sliced medium sweet potato

- 4 Cups of baby spinach
- ½ Cup of beef or vegetable broth
- 1 Cup of sliced almonds
- 1/8 Teaspoon of sea salt
- 1/8 Teaspoon of ground black pepper

Directions:

1. Preheat your oven to about 350°F.
2. Heat a little bit of olive oil into a large non-stick skillet; then add the onion and sauté it until it becomes tender
3. Add in the garlic and cook altogether for 1 additional minute
4. Season with a little bit of salt and pepper; then remove from the pan
5. Add in the beef to your pan; then cook it until it is no longer pink.
6. Season with a little bit of salt and 1 pinch of pepper
7. Add a little bit of Italian seasoning; then turn off the heat
8. Start by spreading a layer of the sweet potatoes into the bottom of a square baking tray
9. Top with the onions, the spinach and the beef; then continue the process of layering your ingredients until you are done with all your ingredients
10. Drizzle with a little quantity of broth; then cover with an aluminium foil paper
11. Bake your tray in the oven for about 30 minutes; then remove it from the oven and sprinkle it with a little bit of almonds.
12. Bake your beef tray for about 10 additional minutes or until the almonds get a brown colour
13. Remove the tray from the oven; then serve and enjoy!

Nutritional information

- Calories per serving – 166.4 calories
- Fat per serving – 4.2 grams
- Saturated Fat – 1.5 gram
- Total Carbs per serving – 18.4 grams
- Protein per serving – 13 grams

ONION BEEF STEW

- *Cooking Time: 50 minutes*
- *Preparation Time: 15 minutes*
- *Servings: 4-5*

- **NOTE:**

This stew recipe is very simple with a few ingredients like tomatoes and beef. You don't need to be a master chef to make the most delicious beef stew ever. The addition of basil and dried oregano will make this recipe rich in naturally spicy flavors.

INGREDIENTS

- 2 Tablespoon of coconut oil
- 1 Pound of cubed beef stew meat
- ¾ Cup of beef stock
- 1 Large, diced onion
- 1 Medium; minced garlic clove
- 1 large carrot
- 2 Cans of diced tomatoes

* 2/3 Cup of red wine
* 1 Teaspoon of dried oregano
* 1 Teaspoon of dried basil

Directions:

1. Heat the oil into a large saucepan over a medium high heat and when it becomes hot, add the beef and sauté it on all its sides
2. Remove the beef meat from the pan and set it aside
3. Add about ¼ cup of stock; then with a wooden spoon; scrape any meat bits from the bottom of your saucepan
4. Add the onions and the garlic; then continue cooking for about 3 minutes
5. Add the remaining quantity of the stock, the sautéed beef, the carrots, the tomatoes, the red wine, the oregano and the basil.
6. Cover your ingredients and let it simmer over a low heat for about 50 minutes
7. Remove the stew from the heat; then serve and enjoy!

Nutritional information

* Calories per serving – 232 calories
* Fat per serving – 7.2 grams
* Saturated Fat – 1.4 gram
* Total Carbs per serving –25.8 grams
* Protein per serving – 17.1grams

Recipe 33: Beef Meatballs
(Cooking Time: 50 minutes \ Preparation Time: 15 minutes \ Servings: 4-5)

* **NOTE:**

What is better than enjoying the combination of two irresistible tastes? How about making a simple dish packed with nutrients and healthy ingredients. This recipe won't cause any rise in the level of sugar within our blood. It is an extremely delicious recipe that everyone will like.

INGREDIENTS

- 1 and ½ pounds of ground beef;
- 1 large egg
- 2 Tablespoons of old fashioned mustard
- 1 Tablespoon of coconut aminos;
- 1 Teaspoon of onion powder
- Coconut oil
- Minced fresh parsley
- 1 Pinch of Sea salt
- 1 Pinch of ground black pepper
- Ingredients to make the gravy
- 1 Chopped onion
- 1 Cup of beef stock
- 2 Tablespoons of clarified coconut oil
- 1 Pinch of Sea salt and 1 pinch of freshly ground black pepper
- Ingredients to make the mashed potatoes:
- 4 Large peeled and chopped sweet potatoes
- 3 Tablespoons of clarified butter
- 1 Pinch of sea salt and 1 pinch of freshly ground black pepper

Directions:

1. Start by cooking the potatoes and boil it in hot water for about 14 to 15 minutes
2. After draining the potatoes; mash it with a potato masher and add the coconut oil; then season it with 1 pinch of

black pepper and 1 pinch of salt

3. In a medium deep bowl, mix the ground beef, the egg; the mustard, the coconut aminos and the onion powder; then season your ingredients with a little bit of salt and with 1 pinch of ground black pepper

4. Shape your meat mixture into the form of meatballs with both your hands.

5. Melt a little bit of coconut oil into a large skillet over a medium heat

6. Toss the meatballs into the skillet; then cook it for a few minutes

7. Remove your meatballs from the skillet and set it aside

8. Without removing the skillet off the heat, add a little bit of coconut oil; then toss in the onion and sauté for a few minutes

9. Pour in the beef stock and return your meatballs to the same skillet; then gently add the gravy

10. Serve your meatballs with the seasoned and mashed potatoes; then top with fresh parsley

11. Serve and enjoy!

Nutritional information

- Calories per serving – 271.1 calories
- Fat per serving – 11.9 grams
- Saturated Fat – 1gram
- Total Carbs per serving – 12.1 grams
- Protein per serving – 27grams

BEEF CHILLI

- ***Cooking Time: 40 minutes***
- ***Preparation Time: 10 minutes***
- ***Servings: 3-4***

- **NOTE:**

A healthy and nutritious meal, this beef chilli recipe makes a perfect choice to help any illness disappear right immediately. This recipe is rich in veggies and packed with proteins and vitamins. There is nothing better than enjoying this beef chilli for a lunch or dinner. Besides, making beef chilli is not a hard job.

INGREDIENTS:

- 1 and ½ pounds of ground beef
- 2 Chopped garlic cloves garlic, chopped
- 2 Tablespoons of coconut oil
- 1 and ½ cups of diced onion
- ½ Cup of chopped celery

- 1 and ½ cups of peeled and cut carrots
- 2 Tablespoons of chilli powder
- 1 Teaspoon of ground cumin
- 1 Teaspoon of oregano
- 1 Teaspoon of salt
- ¼ teaspoon of cayenne pepper
- 4 Cups of diced zucchinis
- 1 Can of 15 oz tomato puree
- 1 Can of diced tomatoes

Directions:

1. In a large and non-stick skillet, season the beef with salt and pepper; then add the garlic and sauté the beef for a few minutes
2. Add the oil, the onions, the celery, the carrots, and the seasonings to your skillet; then cook your ingredients altogether until it becomes translucent over a medium high heat for about 6 minutes
3. Once the onions become golden; add the zucchini and cook altogether for about 2 additional minutes
4. Let your ingredients, simmer for about 20 minutes over a medium heat
5. Add the cooked beef, the tomato puree and the tomatoes into the saucepan; then stir very well
6. Reduce the heat and let you ingredients, simmer for 15 additional minutes
7. Serve and enjoy your chilli!

Nutritional information

- Calories per serving – 249 calories
- Fat per serving – 11.48 grams

- Saturated Fat – 5.5 grams
- Total Carbs per serving –8.9 grams
- Protein per serving – 27.1 grams

SWEET POTATO MEATLOAF

- ***Cooking Time: 60 minutes***
- ***Preparation Time: 15 minutes***
- ***Servings: 5-6***

- **NOTE:**

This Meatloaf is one of the most delicious recipes you can taste with a Paleo twist. You can serve this meatloaf with a mushroom salsa or with a simple salad recipe. You can also enjoy eating a meatloaf with a salad of your choice.

INGREDIENTS

- 2 Pounds of grass-fed ground beef
- 1 Large diced onion
- 1 Cup of cooked sweet potato
- 1 Cup of almond flour
- 2 Tablespoons of coconut flour
- 1 Large egg
- 1 Cup of Paleo ketchup

- 3 Tablespoons of coconut aminos
- 2 Teaspoons of salt
- 1 Teaspoon of garlic powder
- For the glaze
- ½ Cup of Paleo ketchup
- 2 Tablespoons of coconut aminos
- 1 Tablespoon of honey

Directions:

1. Preheat your oven to about 350° and prepare a baking tray by lining it with a cookie sheet or a parchment paper
2. Put the diced onion with a little bit of coconut oil in a saucepan; then sauté it until it becomes soft for about 6 minutes
3. In a large and deep bowl; mix altogether the beef, the onion, the sweet potato, the almond flour, the coconut flour, the egg, the ketchup, the coconut aminos, the salt, and the garlic powder together.
4. Make the form of a loaf and put it into a pan; then mix all the ingredients of the glaze in a bowl and pour it over the meatloaf
5. Bake your meatloaf for about 60 minutes; then remove it from the oven.
6. Set the meatloaf aside to cool; then slice it, serve and enjoy it!

Nutritional information

- Calories per serving – 285 calories
- Fat per serving – 14.02 grams
- Saturated Fat – 3.45 grams
- Total Carbs per serving – 10.7 grams
- Protein per serving – 29.8 grams

BEEF STUFFED MIGNON

- ***Cooking Time: 10 minutes***
- ***Preparation Time: 5 minutes***
- ***Servings: 3***

- **NOTE:**

Do you want to enjoy a great beef lunch; then you should choose a good quality beef filet mignon. This recipe is very unique and rich in vitamins; it will make you feel full because it is packed with proteins and nutrients; you are going to enjoy this recipe for sure.

INGREDIENTS

- 2 Beef filet mignon
- 4 to 5 Pieces of bacon
- ⅛ Teaspoon of garlic powder
- 1 Pinch of salt
- 1 Pinch of black pepper
- 2 Tablespoons of mustard
- 1 Tablespoon of raw honey

- 1 Tablespoon of orange juice

Directions:

1. Preheat your oven to about 375 degrees.
2. Wrap each of the beef filet mignon with the pieces of the bacon so that you cover all the parts of the sides of the beef filet mignon.
3. Secure the filets of the beef mignon with the help of toothpicks and sprinkle a little bit of garlic powder, a little bit of salt and 1 pinch of black pepper
4. Put a large saucepan over a medium high heat; then put each of the filets mignon and sauté it until it is perfectly cooked
5. Sear both of the tops and the bottoms of the fillets for about 3 minutes over each side
6. Transfer the mignon to the oven and add to it the mustard, the honey and the orange juice
7. Once cooked, serve and enjoy your dish!

Nutritional information

- Calories per serving – 246.1 calories
- Fat per serving – 11 grams
- Saturated Fat – 3 grams
- Total Carbs per serving –0 grams
- Protein per serving – 35.9 grams

Recipe 37: Beef burgers
(Cooking Time: 15 minutes \ Preparation Time: 10 minutes \ Servings: 2)

- **NOTE**:

Who said the burgers don't make a healthy choice? Don't worry anymore because this burger recipe is one of the healthiest recipes you can ever taste. Beef burgers are topped with onions and slices of avocado.

INGREDIENTS:

- 1 and ½ pounds of ground beef meat
- 1 Pinch of sea salt
- 1 Teaspoon of ground black pepper
- ½ Tablespoon of garlic powder
- 2 Tablespoons of olive oil or coconut oil
- 2 Small thinly sliced onions
- 1 and ½ tablespoons of balsamic vinegar
- 1 Large sliced tomato beef steak
- Cup of shredded green leaf lettuce
- 2 Avocados

Directions:

1. Place a non-stick medium skillet over a medium high heat.
2. Add 1 tablespoon of the coconut oil; then when it melts; sauté it until it becomes caramelized
3. Add the balsamic vinegar and sauté for about 5 minutes; keep stirring
4. Form about burgers out of the ground beef
5. Season the burgers with a little bit of pepper and with 1 pinch of salt
6. Heat a non-stick skillet over a medium heat and sauté the burgers for about 4 minutes
7. Remove the burgers from the skillet and set it aside for about 1 minute
8. Assemble the burgers by placing the 1 slice of tomato

beef steak over a plate, then top it with the lettuce, your burger and about 2 tablespoons of the onion
9. Top with avocado slices and serve your burgers
10. Enjoy!

Nutritional information

- Calories per serving – 365 calories
- Fat per serving – 26 grams
- Saturated Fat – 8 grams
- Total Carbs per serving –8.1 grams
- Protein per serving – 24.2 grams

SPICY BEEF ROAST WITH PAPRIKA

- ***Cooking Time: 45 minutes***
- ***Preparation Time: 15 minutes***
- ***Servings: 3-4***

- **NOTE:**

An easy to make beef roast with a flavourful gravy, this recipe is very nutritious and healthy. The addition of spices like paprika, garlic and black pepper adds a special twist to your dish.

INGREDIENTS

- 2 Pounds of beef roast
- ½ Teaspoon of sea salt
- ½ Teaspoon of black pepper
- 1 Teaspoon of smoked paprika
- ½ Teaspoon of garlic powder
- 1 Teaspoon of thyme
- ½ Teaspoon of onion powder
- 1 Tablespoon of avocado oil

- 1 and ½ cups of beef broth
- ½ Cup of white wine
- 3 Minced garlic cloves
- 1 and ½ teaspoons of arrowroot powder
- 1 and ½ teaspoons of cold water

Directions:

1. In a bowl, combine altogether the sea salt, the black pepper, the paprika, the garlic powder, the thyme, and the onion powder; then mix very well
2. Rub the seasoning mixture over the roast.
3. Now, heat a saucepan over a high heat and add about 1 tablespoon of oil.
4. Sear the roast on both its sides; then pour the beef broth and the wine over your roast.
5. Sprinkle the minced garlic on top of the garlic; then reduce the heat and let simmer for about 40 minutes
6. Remove the roast from the pot; meanwhile, combine the arrowroot powder with the cold water and stir very well
7. Bring the water and the arrowroot to a boil and let it thicken before pouring it over your sliced roast
8. Serve and enjoy!

Nutritional information

- Calories per serving – 289 calories
- Fat per serving – 17.5 grams
- Saturated Fat – 6.1 grams
- Total Carbs per serving –2 grams
- Protein per serving – 25.9 grams

HONEY GLAZED BEEF WITH BROCCOLI AND CASHEWS

- *Cooking Time: 35 minutes*
- *Preparation Time: 5 minutes*
- *Servings: 3*

- **NOTE:**

How about a delicious dish that melts in your mouth with the taste of beef meat? This dish remains one of the most luxurious and easiest dishes that you can make and serve on any special occasions. And in addition to its delicious taste, this recipe is packed with proteins and vitamins.

INGREDIENTS:

- 1 Cup of coconut aminos
- ½ Cup of orange juice
- 3 Tablespoons of honey
- 1 Teaspoon of fish sauce
- 2 Minced garlic cloves

- 1 Teaspoons of fresh grated ginger
- ½ Teaspoon of red pepper flakes
- 3 Tablespoons of arrowroot powder
- 1 Pound of thinly sliced flank steak
- 3 Cups of broccoli florets
- 1 Pinch of salt and 1 pinch of pepper
- 2 Tablespoons of coconut oil
- ½ Cup of toasted cashews

Directions:

1. Whisk altogether the coconut amines, the orange juice, the honey, the fish sauce, the garlic, the ginger, the red pepper flakes, the arrowroot powder, and 1 Pinch of salt with 1 pinch of pepper.
2. Place the sliced flank steak into a shallow bowl; then pour the whisked mixture over the meat and refrigerate it for about 30 minutes
3. Put a baking tray over a medium heat and add to it 1 tablespoon of coconut oil
4. Add the broccoli florets to the tray and season with salt and pepper
5. Add 1 tablespoon of water and let steam for about 1 minute
6. Remove the broccoli from the tray and set it aside
7. Cook the meat in the same tray and once it becomes brown, add the broccoli and the cashews
8. Mix your ingredients together very well and cook for 1 additional minute
9. Serve and enjoy!

Nutritional information

- Calories per serving – 330 calories

- Fat per serving – 16.6 grams
- Saturated Fat – 4.4 grams
- Total Carbs per serving – 13.9 grams
- Protein per serving – 31.8 grams

- Fat per serving – 16.6 grams
- Saturated Fat – 4.4 grams
- Total Carbs per serving – 13.9 grams
- Protein per serving – 31.8 grams

BEEF STEAK IN ALUMINIUM PAPER

- *Cooking Time: 25 minutes*
- *Preparation Time: 10 minutes*
- *Servings: 3-4*

- **NOTE:**

This butter; Garlic Herb beef Steak, baked in Foil will melt in your mouth as soon as you taste it; and for the first time, you will feel that you can finish the entire dish by yourself. The addition of veggies will enrich your lunch and will add a touch of perfection to it.

INGREDIENTS

- 1 Pound of small red potatoes
- 2 Sliced carrots
- 1 Cubed red bell pepper
- 1 Cubed green bell pepper
- ½ Chopped red onion
- 1 Pinch of salt

- 1 Pinch of pepper
- 1 Tablespoon of olive oil
- 1 and ½ pounds of cubed top sirloin steak
- To make the Garlic Herb Butter use:
- ½ Cup of almond butter to the room temperature
- ¼ Cup of freshly chopped parsley
- 4 Minced garlic cloves
- 1 Teaspoon of chopped fresh rosemary
- 1 Teaspoon of chopped fresh thyme
- ½ Teaspoon of salt
- ¼ Teaspoon of pepper

Directions:

1. In a bowl of medium size, put the red potatoes, the carrots, the bell peppers, and the red onion. Then add the salt and the ground pepper and toss everything together with the olive oil
2. Prepare an aluminium foil paper and put it over a counter
3. Place the vegetables in the foil and top it with the steak.
4. Now, time to prepare the butter of garlic: take a small bowl and put in it the parsley, the almond butter, the garlic, the rosemary, the thyme, the salt and the pepper.
5. Divide the garlic batter and pour it evenly over the steak; then fold the top and the ends of the piece
6. Put the packet over the aluminium on top of the grill and grill it for about 15 minutes
7. Serve and enjoy your lunch!

Nutritional information

- Calories per serving – 302.4 calories

- Fat per serving – 8.01 grams
- Saturated Fat – 0.6 grams
- Total Carbs per serving – 1.2 grams
- Protein per serving – 34.7 grams

SEAFOOD LUNCH RECIPES

BAKED FLOUNDER FILLET

- *Cooking Time: 15 minutes*
- *Preparation Time: 5 minutes*
- *Servings: 2-3*

- **NOTE:**

Have you ever tried this flounder fish recipe? It is one of the most delicious recipes that you can taste; flounder fish is known as a healthy and very nutritious type of fish; you will enjoy it and once you try it, you won't be able to stop making it your daily dish.

INGREDIENTS

- The juice of 1 lemon or lime
- ½ Cup of extra virgin olive oil
- ½ Cup of unsalted melted coconut oil
- 2 Thinly sliced shallots
- 3 Thinly sliced garlic cloves
- 2 Tablespoons of capers

- 1 Teaspoon of seasoned salt
- Teaspoon of ground black pepper
- 1 Teaspoon of ground cumin
- 1 Teaspoon of garlic powder
- 1 and ½ pounds of flounder
- 5 Trimmed green onions from the top; cut the onion lengthwise
- 1 Sliced lime or lemon
- ¾ Cup of chopped fresh dill

Directions:

1. In a small bowl, mix altogether the olive oil with the melted coconut oil
2. Season with a little bit of the seasoned salt and add the shallots, the garlic and the capers.
3. In a separate bowl; mix the seasoned salt with the pepper, the cumin and the garlic powder.
4. Spice the fish fillets, each on both its sides.
5. Put the fish fillets into a greased large baking tray; then cover with the mixture of lime that you have already prepared.
6. Arrange the onion halves and the limes right on top
7. Bake your dish in the oven for about 15 minutes at a heat of about 375° F
8. Remove the fish from your oven and garnish it with toppings of your choice; but first don't forget to garnish with the fresh dill.
9. Serve and enjoy with a salad of your choice.

Nutritional information

- Calories per serving – 142.1 calories

- Fat per serving – 3.90 grams
- Saturated Fat – 0.8 grams
- Total Carbs per serving –0.4 grams
- Protein per serving – 24.7 grams

GARLIC SHRIMP WITH COCONUT MILK

- ***Cooking Time: 15 minutes***
- ***Preparation Time: 5 minutes***
- ***Servings: 2-3***

- **NOTE:**

This garlic shrimp dish is very easy to make and doesn't need many ingredients. In addition to its high nutritional value, this recipe is low in saturated fat and it will help you lose weight in a short time. It is a great recipe if you are busy to make on the go.

INGREDIENTS

- 1 Pound of shrimp
- 1 Tablespoon of melted coconut oil
- 1/8 Teaspoon of chilli flakes
- 3 Tablespoons of chopped garlic
- 2 Tablespoons of canned coconut milk
- 2 Teaspoons of dried parsley
- 1 and ½ Teaspoons of paprika

- ½ Teaspoon of salt
- ½ Teaspoon of ground black pepper
- 2 Tablespoon of lemon juice

Directions:

1. In a large skillet, mix 1 tablespoon of melted coconut oil, 3 tablespoons of garlic, 1/8 teaspoon of chilli flakes and sauté for about 3 minutes
2. Toss the shrimp into the pan; then add 2 tablespoons of coconut milk
3. Add 2 teaspoons of dried parsley, 1 and ½ teaspoons of paprika, ½ teaspoon of salt
4. Add ½ teaspoon of ground black pepper, and 2 tablespoons of lemon juice.
5. Cook the shrimp for about 9 minutes
6. Transfer the shrimp to a platter and make the sauce in the skillet; then return the shrimp to the pan and mix it with the sauce
7. Serve and enjoy your dish!

Nutritional information

- Calories per serving – 210.4 calories
- Fat per serving – 1.35 grams
- Saturated Fat – 0.8 grams
- Total Carbs per serving –3.5 grams
- Protein per serving – 31.1 grams

OVEN BAKED SALMON FILLETS

- ***Cooking Time: 10 minutes***
- ***Preparation Time: 4 minutes***
- ***Servings: 3-4***

- **NOTE:**

This delicious and simple fish recipe combines the crusty textures of the succulent salmon fillets with a Paleo twist. You don't need any sophisticated ingredients to cook this salmon crusted dish. It is light, simple, and incredibly succulent.

INGREDIENTS:

- About 2 salmon fillets of 6oz each
- 1 Tablespoon of coconut flour
- 2 Tablespoons of fresh parsley
- 1 Tablespoon of olive oil
- 1 Tablespoon of Dijon mustard
- 1 Pinch of salt
- 1 Pinch of pepper

- To make the salad
- 2 Cups of arugula
- ¼ Thinly sliced red onion
- The juice of 1 lemon
- 1 Tablespoon of white wine vinegar
- 1 Tablespoon of olive oil
- 1 Pinch of salt and 1 pinch of ground black pepper

Directions:

1. Preheat your oven to about 450°F.
2. Place the salmon fillets over a parchment lined baking sheet.
3. Top the salmon with a drizzle of olive oil ad with Dijon mustard; then rub the spices into the salmon.
4. In a small and deep bowl, mix altogether the coconut flour, the parsley, and the salt
5. Add 1 pinch of pepper.
6. With a spoon; spread the mixture over the salmon fillets; then bake for about 10 minutes; in the meantime, prepare the salad by mixing all the ingredients of the salad
7. Remove the salmon from the oven and serve it with the salad
8. Enjoy!

Nutritional information

- Calories per serving – 259.1 calories
- Fat per serving – 14.2 grams
- Saturated Fat – 4.2 gram
- Total Carbs per serving – 7.3 grams
- Protein per serving – 24.3 grams

SALMON WITH MUSHROOMS

- ***Cooking Time: 12 minutes***
- ***Preparation Time: 5 minutes***
- ***Servings: 3***

- **NOTE:**

What is better than a quick salmon dish prepared with extra care for a delicious lunch? You will enjoy the taste of salmon and the combination of salmon with the mushrooms adds a special and unique flavourful taste to your dish.

INGREDIENTS

- 2 tablespoons of cooking spray
- 3 to 4 salmon fillets of about 1 inch of thickness
- ½ Teaspoon of salt, divided
- ¼ Teaspoon of black pepper
- 1 Teaspoon of olive oil
- 1 Tablespoon thinly sliced shallots
- 1 and ½ cups of Presliced mushrooms

- 2 Cups of fresh spinach
- 1 Teaspoon of grated lemon rind
- 1 Teaspoon of fresh lemon juice

Directions:

1. Start by heating a large non-stick skillet and coat it with a little bit of cooking spray over a medium-high heat.
2. Sprinkle the fish with about ¼ teaspoon of salt and ground pepper.
3. Add the fish to the pan; then cook for about 5 minutes
4. Remove the fish from the pan, and keep it warm.
5. Add the oil and the shallots to the pan; then sauté for about 1 minute.
6. Add the mushrooms and layer it into 1 layer
7. Cook for about 2 minutes and stir from time to time
8. Add the spinach and cook it for about 30 seconds
9. Remove the spinach from the heat and add ¼ teaspoon of salt, the rind and the juice
10. Serve the fish with lemon rinds
11. Enjoy!

Nutritional information

- Calories per serving – 297.9 calories
- Fat per serving – 14.3 grams
- Saturated Fat – 3.2 gram
- Total Carbs per serving –2.9 grams
- Protein per serving – 37.7 grams

TILAPIA BITES

- *Cooking Time: 20 minutes*
- *Preparation Time: 10 minutes*
- *Servings: 8*

- **NOTE:**

There are many ways in which you can enjoy the taste of tilapia and one of which is to enjoy the incredible delicious taste of these fish bites. This is a different approach that can help you enjoy a new recipe that you might have never tasted. In addition to its tastiness, no one can ignore the nutritious taste of tilapia bites.

INGREDIENTS

- 1 and 1/3 pounds of tilapia or 6 filets
- ¼ Cup of lemon juice
- 2 Large eggs
- 1 Teaspoon of onion powder
- 1 Teaspoon of garlic powder
- 1 Teaspoon of fresh thyme

- 1 Tablespoon of horseradish mustard
- ½ Teaspoon of salt
- ¼ Teaspoon of black pepper
- 1 and ½ cups of almond flour
- 1 and ½ tablespoons of olive oil

Directions:

1. Preheat your oven to about 400° F.
2. Line a cookie sheet with aluminium foil and grease the aluminium foil with a little bit of oil
3. Put the tilapia filets over the top of the aluminium foil and cook it for about 20 minutes.
4. Once the tilapia is ready; remove it from the oven and break it with forks into pieces
5. In another bowl, combine the lemon juice with the eggs, the onion powder, the garlic powder, the mustard, the salt, the pepper, and the thyme
6. Toss in the fish with about ½ cup of the almond flour and mix very well with the use of a fork
7. Place about 1 cup of almond flour over a platter.
8. With about ¼ cup of a measuring scoop, form patties from the mixture in your hand
9. Dip both the top and the bottom of the patties into the mixture of the almond flour; then put the line the fish patties over a platter
10. Put the patties in the refrigerator for about 30 minutes
11. Heat about 1 tablespoon of olive oil into a large skillet over a medium-high heat.
12. Cook each of the fish patties for about 4 minutes, then flip it and cook it for about 3 minutes.
13. Remove the patties from the skillet and put it over a paper towel
14. Serve and enjoy!

Nutritional information

- Calories per serving – 285.1 calories
- Fat per serving – 16.6 grams
- Saturated Fat – 4.2 gram
- Total Carbs per serving –4.5 grams
- Protein per serving – 27.7 grams

TUNA SALAD

- ***Cooking Time: 5 minutes***
- ***Preparation Time: 5 minutes***
- ***Servings: 3***

- **NOTE:**

This salad is a very easy and quick-to make recipe. There are many veggies that you can add to this tuna salad. It is a healthy and a great salad recipe to enjoy for a light lunch and to serve a perfect Paleo lunch. You will feel full and at the same time you will feel energized with this salad.

INGREDIENTS

- 1 Can of white drained Albacore Tuna
- ½ Large, diced red bell pepper
- ½ Peeled and cut large carrot
- ¼ Cup of diced grape tomatoes
- 1 Thinly sliced scallion; only use the green part
- 1 Small mashed avocado

- 1 Tablespoon of lemon juice
- ½ Teaspoon of fine grain sea salt

Directions:

1. In a large bowl, mix altogether the diced veggies, the tuna, the mashed avocado, the lime juice, the sliced scallions and the salt until your ingredients are very well combined.
2. Serve your tuna salad with a wrap
3. Enjoy this delicious tuna salad or store it in the refrigerator and enjoy it later!

Nutritional information

- Calories per serving – 142.1 calories
- Fat per serving – 8.0 grams
- Saturated Fat – 0.8 gram
- Total Carbs per serving – 5.3 grams
- Protein per serving – 11.8 grams

BAKED COD WITH SWEET POTATOES

- ***Cooking Time: 30 minutes***
- ***Preparation Time: 5 minutes***
- ***Servings: 4***

- **NOTE:**

This sweet potatoes and fish dish is very good for anyone to remain healthy and sane. The combination of fish with zucchini will let you enjoy a crisp taste that you will never forget. Besides, this recipe is quick and will help you lose weight.

INGREDIENTS:

- 1 Tablespoon of paprika
- 1 Tablespoon of smoked paprika
- ½ Teaspoon of cumin
- ½ Teaspoon of oregano
- ½ Teaspoon of garlic powder
- ½ Teaspoon of salt

- ¼ Teaspoon of coriander
- ¼ Teaspoon of black pepper
- 1/8 Teaspoon of cayenne pepper
- 1 Tablespoon of olive oil
- 4 Chopped sweet potatoes
- 1 and ½ pounds of cod filets
- 1 Chopped zucchini
- 1 Chopped summer squash
- 6 Oz of fish
- 1 and ½ cups of veggies

Directions

1. Preheat your oven to about 400° F.
2. Mix your ingredients together with the spices in order to create the seasoning
3. Add the sweet potatoes with the olive oil and with half of the seasoning mixture
4. Line a baking sheet with aluminium foil and grease it with cooking spray
5. Layer the potatoes over the baking sheet and put it in the oven for about 20 minutes
6. After about 20 minutes, add the zucchini, the fish and the summer squash.
7. Sprinkle with a little bit of blackening seasoning.
8. Return the baking tray to the oven and cook it for about 10 minutes
9. Serve and enjoy your dish!

Nutritional information

- Calories per serving – 302 calories
- Fat per serving – 5.1 grams

- Saturated Fat – 1.1 gram
- Total Carbs per serving –32 grams
- Protein per serving – 34 grams

COD FISH WITH TOMATO SAUCE

- ***Cooking Time: 30 minutes***
- ***Preparation Time: 5 minutes***
- ***Servings: 4***

- **NOTE:**

Can you think of a taste better than the cod filets with the tomato sauce? You will like the flavourful taste of cod combined with the white wine and the tomato sauce; it is very beneficial and nutritional too.

INGREDIENTS

- To make the Tomato Basil Sauce:
- 2 Tablespoons of olive oil
- ½ Teaspoon of crushed red pepper flakes
- 2 Large, finely minced garlic cloves
- 1 Sliced pint of cherry tomatoes
- ¼ Cup of dry white wine
- ½ Cup of finely chopped fresh basil

- 2 Tablespoons of fresh lemon juice
- ½ Teaspoon of fresh lemon zest
- ½ Teaspoon of salt
- ¼ Teaspoon of fresh ground black pepper
- To prepare the Cod:
- 2 Tablespoons of olive oil
- 1 and ½ pounds of fresh and cut cod
- 1 Pinch of salt and 1 pinch of pepper

Directions:

1. Preheat your oven to about 375° F
2. To make the White Wine Tomato Basil Sauce:
3. Heat the oil in a large pan over a medium heat
4. Add the crushed red pepper flakes and the garlic; then sauté the ingredients altogether for about 1 to 2 minutes
5. Add the tomatoes and cook the ingredients for about 13 minutes; but make sure to stir from time to time
6. Pour in the white wine and let simmer; then add the basil, the lemon juice, the lemon zest, the salt and the pepper and cook for about 2 minutes
7. Transfer your sauce to a medium bowl; then set it aside
8. To make the Cod:
9. Heat the oil in a large skillet and sauté it over a medium heat.
10. Season both the sides of the Cod with the salt and the pepper.
11. Put the cod into the oil and cook it for about 4 minutes
12. Flip the cod from time to time and bake it in the oven for about 5 minutes
13. Pour the wine over the tomato basil sauce and serve it.
14. Enjoy your lunch!

Nutritional information

- Calories per serving – 163.3 calories
- Fat per serving – 4.2 grams
- Saturated Fat – 0.7 gram
- Total Carbs per serving –4.3 grams
- Protein per serving – 21 grams

SCALLOPS WITH GARLIC

- ***Cooking Time: 8 minutes***
- ***Preparation Time: 4 minutes***
- ***Servings: 3***

- **NOTE:**

Do you want to enjoy a scrumptious dish rich in various flavours? Then don't wait any longer and make this scallop recipe with great care and perfection. It is a healthy and great choice to serve for lunch or dinner. This dish is one of the best dishes par excellence.

INGREDIENTS

- 1 Pound of large scallops
- ¼ Cups of clarified ghee
- 5 Grated garlic cloves
- 1 Large zest of lemon
- ¼ Cup of chopped Italian parsley
- ½ Teaspoon of sea salt

- ¼ Teaspoon of freshly ground peppercorn
- ¼ Teaspoon of red pepper flakes
- 1 pinch of sweet paprika
- 1 Teaspoon of extra virgin olive oil

Directions:

1. Start by patting dry all of your scallops with a paper towel very well.
2. Heat a non-stick skillet over a medium heat
3. Put the scallops with a little bit of olive oil and sprinkle it with a little bit of sea salt, a little bit of cracked pepper, the red pepper flakes and with sweet paprika.
4. Toss the scallops to coat it and add a little bit of ghee to your hot skillet
5. Add in the scallops to the pan and sear it for about 3 minutes
6. Add the ghee to your skillet and the scallops; then stir in the garlic and remove the ingredients from the heat
7. Squeeze half of your lemon on top of the scallops.
8. Garnish with parsley and lemon zest
9. Serve and enjoy!

Nutritional information

- Calories per serving – 181.3 calories
- Fat per serving – 14.4 grams
- Saturated Fat – 2.7 gram
- Total Carbs per serving – 14.3 grams
- Protein per serving – 1.8 grams

Recipe 50: Coconut crusted Shrimp
(Cooking Time: 10 minutes \ Preparation Time: 5 minutes \ Servings: 5)

- **NOTE:**

These crunchy shrimp are a perfect and light seafood dish that you are going to like very much. It is a dish rich in proteins and in vitamins. There is nothing better for seafood lovers than enjoying this recipe.

INGREDIENTS

- 1 and ½ pounds of large peeled and deveined shrimps
- 2 Large eggs
- ¼ Teaspoon of black pepper
- ½ Teaspoon of salt
- 2 Cups of unsweetened shredded coconut
- Coconut oil for frying

Directions:

1. In a medium shallow bowl, crack in the eggs and beat it with the salt and the black pepper; then set it aside
2. Put the shredded coconut into a large plate.
3. Dip each of the shrimps into the egg wash; then press each shrimp into the coconut
4. Now, pour the coconut oil into a large non-stick skillet over a medium heat
5. Fry your shrimps for about 3 to 4 minutes per batch
6. Serve the shrimp with your favourite sauce
7. Enjoy!

Nutritional information

- Calories per serving – 309 calories
- Fat per serving – 16.9 grams
- Saturated Fat – 4.9 gram
- Total Carbs per serving –28.1 grams

- Protein per serving – 13.9 grams

CHAPTER 4

SIDE DISHES

GARLIC BAKED MUSHROOMS

- ***Cooking Time: 9 minutes***
- ***Preparation Time: 3 minutes***
- ***Servings: 4-5***

- **NOTE:**

THIS SIDE DISH of these garlic sautéed mushrooms makes one of the best mushroom dishes you can serve and make. It is a delicious recipe to make on special occasions. It is not only a simple recipe, but also rich in flavours.

INGREDIENTS:

- 1 Pound of white button mushrooms
- 3 Tablespoons of bacon fat
- 1 Small, finely chopped white onion
- 2 Chopped garlic cloves garlic
- ½ Teaspoon of sea salt
- ¼ Teaspoon of ground black pepper
- 1 and ½ tablespoons of balsamic vinegar

- 1 Tablespoon of chopped fresh parsley

Directions:

1. Start by cleaning and wiping your mushrooms gently with a damp paper; then slice each one in halves and set it aside
2. Put the bacon fat in a large non-stick skillet over a medium heat
3. Add in the mushrooms, the onion and the garlic; then cook for about 9 minutes
4. Cook the mushrooms until it becomes tender and stir through the process
5. Season with the sea salt, the pepper and the balsamic vinegar; then stir very well to combine your ingredients.
6. Cook for about 2 minutes; then garnish with parsley
7. Serve and enjoy!

Nutritional information

- Calories per serving – 193.5 calories
- Fat per serving – 13.8 grams
- Saturated Fat – 6.4 gram
- Total Carbs per serving –3.8 grams
- Protein per serving – 13.5 grams

ALMOND FLOUR SCONES

- ***Cooking Time: 15 minutes***
- ***Preparation Time: 10 minutes***
- ***Servings: 6***

- **NOTE:**

There is nothing better than the magic herb dough, which helps us to make tender and at the same time flavourful almond flour scones that you will enjoy very much.

INGREDIENTS

- 2 Cups of almond flour
- ¼ Cup of chopped fresh parsley
- 1 Tablespoon of fresh thyme
- 1 Teaspoon of fresh rosemary
- 1 Teaspoon of baking soda
- 1 Teaspoon of sea salt
- Fresh herbs
- 2 large beaten eggs

Directions:

1. Start by preheating your oven to about 375° F.
2. In a large and deep bowl, mix altogether the almond flour with the herbs, the salt and the baking soda. Then mix very well.
3. In another bowl, crack the eggs and whisk it; then add the eggs to the bowl of the dry ingredients and stir very well to form the dough
4. Divide your dough into about 6 portions of equal size.
5. Put the dough over a greased baking sheet; then bake it in the oven for about 11 minutes
6. Serve and enjoy your scones!

Nutritional information

- Calories per serving – 294.8 calories
- Fat per serving – 27.2 grams
- Saturated Fat – 1.1 gram
- Total Carbs per serving –7.4 grams
- Protein per serving – 1.4 grams

SWEET POTATO BITES

- ***Cooking Time: 10 minutes***
- ***Preparation Time: 5 minutes***
- ***Servings: 5-6***

- **NOTE:**

This is a great side dish and a great substitute for ordinary potato patties. This recipe is incredibly delicious and light too. You can serve this side dish with a salad or with a healthy Paleo lunch too.

INGREDIENTS

- 2 Large, peeled and cubed sweet potatoes
- ¼ Medium, finely diced onion
- 2 Tablespoons of coconut flour
- 1 Teaspoon of garlic powder
- 1 Teaspoon of chili powder
- ½ Teaspoon of salt
- ¼ Teaspoon of freshly ground pepper
- ½ Cup of coconut oil

Directions

1. Put a quantity of water and let it boil for about 5 minutes
2. Toss in the sweet potatoes and cook altogether for 6 minutes
3. Drain the potatoes and rinse it with the cold water
4. Put the potatoes and the onion altogether in a food processor; then pulse it and transfer the potatoes to a bowl
5. Add the coconut flour; the garlic powder, the chili powder, the salt, and the pepper. Then stir very well to combine it.
6. With your hands, shape the mixture of the potatoes into small patties; then set it aside
7. Heat the oil into a heavy skillet until it becomes hot; then fry the sweet potato patties in the oil for about 4 to 5 minutes
8. Put the sweet potato patties over a paper towel lined platter
9. Serve and enjoy!

Nutritional information

- Calories per serving – 210 calories
- Fat per serving – 7.6 grams
- Saturated Fat – 0.5 gram
- Total Carbs per serving – 33 grams
- Protein per serving – 2.2 grams

FRIED EGGPLANTS

- ***Cooking Time: 20 minutes***
- ***Preparation Time: 7 minutes***
- ***Servings: 2***

- **NOTE:**

This recipe is creamy and scrumptious with the crunchy taste of the almond flour. And this recipe is very well-known by the Paleo diet followers; it is delicious and nutritious. Once you make your own eggplant fries; you will love it and you will get addicted to it.

INGREDIENTS

- 1 Medium, sliced eggplant
- 2 Cups of almond meal
- 2 Teaspoons of fresh rosemary
- 1 and ½ teaspoons of dried thyme
- 1 Teaspoon of smoked paprika
- ¾ Teaspoon of salt
- 2 Large eggs

- 2 Tablespoons of extra virgin olive oil
- To make the dipping Sauce:
- ½ Cup of organic mayonnaise
- ¼ Teaspoon of chili powder
- ¼ Teaspoon of smoked paprika
- ¼ Teaspoon of Dijon mustard
- 1 Teaspoon of ketchup

Directions

1. Preheat your oven to about 450° F
2. Line a baking sheet with a parchment paper
3. Stir the almond meal with the rosemary, the thyme, the paprika, and the salt into a large dish.
4. In another dish, mix the egg with the olive oil and dip the eggplant slices into the mixture of the egg
5. Dredge the eggplant slices in the almond flour
6. Place the eggplant slices over the baking sheet; then bake the eggplant fries in the oven for about 20 minutes
7. Serve and enjoy your fries!

Nutritional information

- Calories per serving – 233.6 calories
- Fat per serving – 17.5 grams
- Saturated Fat – 7.2 gram
- Total Carbs per serving –8.6 grams
- Protein per serving – 11.6 grams

ZUCCHINI PATTIES

- *Cooking Time: 25 minutes*
- *Preparation Time: 5 minutes*
- *Servings: 4-5*

- **NOTE:**

These spicy zucchini patties are rich with various flavors. This recipe of zucchini patties won't disappoint you. You will like the natural taste of your nutritious zucchini patties.

INGREDIENTS

- 2 Medium shredded zucchini
- 1 Teaspoon of sea salt
- ¼ Cup of coconut flour
- 1 Beaten egg
- 1 Teaspoon of black pepper
- ¼ Teaspoon of cayenne pepper
- Coconut oil

Directions:

1. Start by shredding the zucchini with a food box grater
2. Place the shredded zucchini in a bowl and Sprinkle with sea salt and black pepper
3. Set the zucchini aside for about 10 minutes
4. Rinse the zucchini and squeeze any moisture
5. Sift in the coconut flour, the egg and the pepper; then stir very well.
6. Heat a non-stick skillet over a medium heat and melt a little bit of coconut oil in it
7. Fill about ¼ cup of the measuring cup with the mixture of zucchini; then press it down in the cup
8. Flip the cup and flatten it until you form a patty
9. Cook the patties on each side for about 5 minutes and repeat the same process with the remaining batter
10. Let the zucchini patties cool aside for about 3 minutes
11. Serve and enjoy your patties

Nutritional information

- Calories per serving – 151.1 calories
- Fat per serving –7.5 grams
- Saturated Fat – 2.1 gram
- Total Carbs per serving –12 grams
- Protein per serving – 10.2 grams

Recipe 56: Zucchini patties

(Cooking Time: 16 minutes \ Preparation Time: 5 minutes \ Servings: 5-6)

- **NOTE:**

This savory dish that has no excessive fats in it; it is fabulous and makes a great alternative to the mashed potatoes. You can enjoy this side dish with lunch or dinner. It is a one hundred percent healthy recipe.

INGREDIENTS

- 1 Bulb of roasted garlic
- 1 Head of cauliflower
- 2 Cups of low-sodium vegetable stock
- 1 Pinch of coarse salt
- 1 Pinch of freshly-ground black pepper
- 2 Tablespoons of diced fresh chives
- 2 Tablespoons of olive oil

Directions:

1. Cut the cauliflower and put it in a large saucepan with 2 cups of stock
2. Let the cauliflower boil for about 16 minutes
3. Remove the boiled cauliflower from the saucepan and put the cauliflower into a food processor
4. Add 2 tablespoons of stock to the cauliflower
5. Season the cauliflower with about 2 tablespoons of stock, olive oil, the roasted garlic, the salt and the pepper
6. Add in the fresh stock and garnish with more chives
7. Serve and enjoy your side dish!

Nutritional information

- Calories per serving – 142.1 calories
- Fat per serving – 10.5 grams
- Saturated Fat – 2.2 gram
- Total Carbs per serving – 8.95 grams
- Protein per serving – 4.8 grams

MASHED SWEET POTATOES

- ***Cooking Time: 25 minutes***
- ***Preparation Time: 5 minutes***
- ***Servings: 4-5***

- **NOTE:**

Get ready to try this Paleo recipe made of sweet potatoes; it makes an incredible side dish to enjoy with any meal. The use of coconut flakes adds a special taste to this dish and the combination of cinnamon and maple syrup adds a sweet taste that you will like.

INGREDIENTS

- 5 large peeled and chopped sweet potatoes
- 3 Tablespoons of ghee
- 3 Tablespoons of maple syrup
- 1 Teaspoon of vanilla extract
- 2 Teaspoons of cinnamon
- 1 Pinch of nutmeg
- 1 Pinch of salt

- 1 Cup of chopped walnuts
- ½ Cup of unsweetened chopped coconut flakes
- 2 Tablespoons of coconut oil

Directions:

1. Fill a large pot with water and let boil for about 12 minutes
2. Toss the potatoes into the boiling water and let simmer for about 10 minutes
3. Remove the potatoes from the heat and let it drain
4. Preheat your oven to about 350° F.
5. Add about 2 tablespoons of maple syrup and ghee to the sweet potatoes; then add the vanilla, 1 teaspoon of cinnamon, the nutmeg and the salt
6. Mash your potatoes with the rest of the ingredients
7. Season with the salt and transfer the mashed potatoes to a serving platter
8. In a separate bowl; mix the coconut flakes with the walnuts, the coconut oil, the ghee and the syrup; then sprinkle with cinnamon
9. Top the sweet potatoes with walnuts and bake it for about 19 minutes
10. Serve and enjoy!

Nutritional information

- Calories per serving – 151 calories
- Fat per serving –3.6 grams
- Saturated Fat – 1 gram
- Total Carbs per serving –27 grams
- Protein per serving – 3 grams

POTATO SALAD

- ***Cooking Time: 30 minutes***
- ***Preparation Time: 10 minutes***
- ***Servings: 3***

- **NOTE:**

This recipe is very easy and makes a perfect Paleo sweet potato side dish to serve with any lunch or dinner. What is special about this potato salad is that is spicy and packed with vegetables.

INGREDIENTS

- 2 Pounds of sweet potatoes
- 1 Pinch of sea salt
- 4 Large beaten eggs
- 1/3 Cup of Pistachios
- 1 and ¼ cups of diced cucumber
- 1 Cup of cubed Roma Tomato
- ½ Cup of roughly chopped Cilantro
- ½ Cup of thinly sliced Dates

- 3 Tablespoons of thinly sliced fresh mint
- Components to prepare the dressing:
- 1 Cup of roasted soaked cashews
- 7 and ½ tablespoons of Water
- 2 Tablespoons and 1 teaspoon of fresh lemon juice
- 1 Tablespoon of Lemon zest
- 2 and ¼ teaspoons of ground cumin
- 2 and ¼ teaspoon of fresh minced ginger
- 1 and ½ teaspoons of ground cinnamon
- 1 Teaspoon of sea salt
- ¼ Teaspoon of Paprika
- ¼ Teaspoon of Ground allspice
- 1 Pinch of pepper

Directions:

1. Rinse and cut the potatoes into small cubes; then put it in a large saucepan and sprinkle with salt
2. Let your ingredients boil over a medium heat and cook for about 20 minutes
3. Drain the potatoes and set it aside to cool
4. Put the eggs into a medium pan and cover it with water; then boil it for about 10 minutes
5. Set the eggs aside to cool; then preheat the oven to about 375° F and toast the pistachios until it becomes golden for about 10 minutes
6. Drain the water from the cashews and put it in a blender
7. Add the rest of the dressing elements and blend altogether until your ingredients becomes smooth
8. Peel the skin of the boiled potatoes; then chop it into cubes of ¾ inch each
9. Add the cucumber, the tomato, the cilantro, the dates, the mint and the chopped pistachios.

10. Peel your eggs and chop it; then add it to the bowl and pour your prepared dressing on top of the salad

Nutritional information

- Calories per serving – 121.7 calories
- Fat per serving –3.1 grams
- Saturated Fat – 0.45 gram
- Total Carbs per serving –18.4 grams
- Protein per serving – 6.1 grams

COCONUT CRUSTED ONION RINGS

- ***Cooking Time: 10 minutes***
- ***Preparation Time: 5 minutes***
- ***Servings: 1-2***

- **NOTE:**

Do you know that the onion has always been used as a natural cleanser and detoxifying ingredients. The sharp and sweet taste of onion gives it its uniqueness. There is absolutely no one who doesn't like eating onion with any dish.

INGREDIENTS

- 1 Onion
- ½ Cup of coconut flour
- ¼ Cup of arrowroot powder
- ½ Teaspoon of garlic powder
- 1 Teaspoon of salt
- ½ Teaspoon of pepper
- 2 Large eggs

- Coconut oil

Directions:

1. Heat the coconut oil over a medium high heat in a large non-stick skillet
2. Mix the coconut flour, the arrowroot and the spices over a large dish
3. Beat the eggs in a large bowl
4. Peel; then thinly slice a whole onion into thin rings
5. Separate the rings, then dip it into the egg mixture and later in the mixture of the coconut
6. Drop the onion rings in the heated oil; then cook it for about 2 to 3 minutes per side
7. Remove the onion and set it aside to cool
8. Serve and enjoy your onion rings!

Nutritional information

- Calories per serving – 141 calories
- Fat per serving – 10 grams
- Saturated Fat – 2.1 gram
- Total Carbs per serving – 9.1 grams
- Protein per serving – 7.1 grams

EGG MAYONNAISE SALAD

- ***Cooking Time: 20 minutes***
- ***Preparation Time: 10 minutes***
- ***Servings: 5-6***

- **NOTE:**

This salad is based on hard boiled eggs, with red onion and Paleo mayonnaise. It is a healthy recipe and no one can resist its delicious and nutritious taste. This recipe is perfect to serve with any lunch and extremely delicious.

INGREDIENTS:

- 10 Boiled eggs
- 5 Crumbled pieces of bacon
- 1 Medium, chopped medium red onion
- Grapes, sliced almonds and raisins

Directions:

1. Start by cooking the bacon; then hard boil the eggs, chop your onion. Then make the mayonnaise
2. Mix all of the ingredients into a large bowl and add the mayonnaise to it.
3. Store the egg side dish in the refrigerator; then serve it with a salad or lunch
4. Enjoy!

Nutritional information

- Calories per serving – 200.6 calories
- Fat per serving – 12.4 grams
- Saturated Fat – 3.8 gram
- Total Carbs per serving – 4.2 grams
- Protein per serving – 17.2 grams

CHAPTER 5

SNACKS AND APPETIZERS

PALEO NUTS BOWL

- ***Cooking Time: 20 minutes***
- ***Preparation Time: 5 minutes***
- ***Servings: 3***

- **NOTE:**

YOU ARE hungry and you can't think of a healthy snack? Here is our suggestion; try this Paleo snack and you will get addicted to it. It is smoky, salty and the taste of garlic is incredible.

INGREDIENTS

- 3 Cups of mixed nuts; walnut, almonds and cashews
- 1 Tablespoon of garlic infused in olive oil
- 1 Teaspoon of smoked sea salt to taste
- 1 Teaspoon of smoked sweet paprika
- ¼ Teaspoon of smoked hot paprika

Directions

1. Preheat your oven to about 325° F.
2. Combine the nuts into a large bowl and drizzle with the olive oil until your ingredients are very-well coated.
3. Combine the salt and the spices into a small bowl.
4. Sprinkle the spices over the nuts and stir very well until your nuts are combined
5. Spread the nuts into one layer over a baking sheet; then bake in the oven for about 20 minutes
6. Serve and enjoy!

Nutritional information

- Calories per serving – 203 calories
- Fat per serving –14.9 grams
- Saturated Fat – 1 gram
- Total Carbs per serving –23 grams
- Protein per serving – 10. 1 grams

TOASTED CASHEWS

- ***Cooking Time: 10 minutes***
- ***Preparation Time: 5 minutes***
- ***Servings: 2***

- **NOTE:**

The taste of toasted cashews is a perfect snack recipe. And not only cashews are characterized by being low in fats; but it is also has many unpredictable protective benefits.

INGREDIENTS:

- 2 Pounds of Raw Cashews
- ¼ Cup of Extra Virgin Coconut Oil
- 1 Tablespoon of Finely Chopped Fresh Rosemary
- 1 Tablespoon of Kosher Salt
- 2 Teaspoon of Hot Paprika
- 2 Teaspoon of Cracked Black Pepper

Directions:

1. Preheat the oven to about 400°F.
2. Line a baking sheet with an aluminum foil paper.
3. Spread the cashews into the baking sheet
4. Bake the cashews for about 9 minutes
5. Melt the coconut oil in a small pot
6. Lower the heat and toss in the seasonings
7. Transfer the cashews to a serving bowl and add your seasoned coconut oil; then stir very well
8. Serve and enjoy!

Nutritional information

- Calories per serving – 162 calories
- Fat per serving – 13.12 grams
- Saturated Fat – 2.56 gram
- Total Carbs per serving – 9.26 grams
- Protein per serving – 4.33 grams

FRIED SPINACH

- *Cooking Time: 11 minutes*
- *Preparation Time: 5 minutes*
- *Servings: 3*

- **NOTE:**

This recipe is not an ordinary recipe of unhealthy fried chips; but it is a unique one as it uses spinach. Spinach is not only a healthy ingredient, but it helps for a better digestion. The taste of spinach is crispy and delicious too.

INGREDIENTS:

- 2 Boxes of 10 Oz each chopped spinach
- 2 Cans of 14 Oz of artichoke hearts
- 1 Tablespoon of extra-virgin olive oil
- 1 Small diced onion
- 2 Minced garlic cloves
- 1 and ½ teaspoons of sea salt
- 1 Teaspoon of onion powder

- ½ Teaspoon of garlic powder
- ½ Teaspoon of black pepper
- ¼ Teaspoon of cayenne pepper
- 1 Tablespoon of lemon juice
- 1 and ½ cups of cashew cream

Directions:

1. Start by defrosting the spinach; then squeeze out any excess of water; then set it aside
2. Drain; then cut the artichokes
3. Pour the olive oil in a pan; then sauté for about 10 minutes with the onion
4. Add the garlic; then cook for about 1 minute
5. Add the artichoke; the salt, the onion powder, the garlic powder, the black pepper and the cayenne; then heat your ingredients.
6. Add the spinach and the lemon juice; then stir very well
7. Add the cashew cream
8. Serve and enjoy!

Nutritional information

- Calories per serving – 116 calories
- Fat per serving –1.9 grams
- Saturated Fat – 0.25 gram
- Total Carbs per serving –20.4 grams
- Protein per serving – 13.1 grams

CAULIFLOWER STICKS WITH BASIL

- ***Cooking Time: 30 minutes***
- ***Preparation Time: 15 minutes***
- ***Servings: 8***

- **NOTE:**

The creative idea of making cauliflower sticks with basil stems from the culinary passion of substituting breadsticks for a healthy alternative. Cauliflower sticks is not only low in carbohydrates, but also low in fats. It is a very delicious snack to enjoy anytime.

INGREDIENTS

- 1 Medium head of cauliflower
- ½ Tablespoon of oregano
- 1 Tablespoon of basil
- 1 Tablespoon of onion powder
- ½ Teaspoon of red pepper flakes
- 2 Large eggs
- 1 Pinch of salt and pepper

Directions

1. Microwave the entire head of cauliflower in a heat proof dish for about 10 minutes
2. Remove the cauliflower from the microwave and pulse it in a food processor until it becomes smooth
3. Refrigerate the cauliflower for about 10 minutes; then combine the remaining ingredients with it
4. Prepare a baking sheet by greasing it with a little bit of oil
5. Press down the cauliflower into the baking sheet until it becomes of about ½ inch of thickness
6. Put the baking sheet in the oven for about 24 minutes and the heat to about 425° F
7. Remove the cauliflower from the oven and set it to a broil at about 500
8. Cut the cauliflower into sticks; then flip it and put it back in the oven and cook it for about 15 minutes
9. Serve and enjoy!

Nutritional information

- Calories per serving – 163 calories
- Fat per serving –9.7 grams
- Saturated Fat – 4.2 gram
- Total Carbs per serving –4.2 grams
- Protein per serving – 15.5 grams

COCONUT GRANOLA

- *Cooking Time: 20 minutes*
- *Preparation Time: 10 minutes*
- *Servings: 5-6*

- **NOTE:**

Whether you adopted a Paleo-diet, a sugar-free diet or any other special diet, this recipe is the healthiest you can find. The use of almonds and cashews is very beneficial for your health; it improves the cardiovascular circulation and protects us from any sudden risk that can affect our health.

INGREDIENTS

- ½ Cup of coconut nectar
- 1/3 Cup of extra virgin olive oil
- 2 Sprigs of rosemary
- 1 Tablespoon of pure vanilla extract
- 1 Teaspoon of fine grain sea salt
- ¼ Teaspoon of cayenne

- 1 Teaspoon of coarsely ground black pepper
- 1 Cup of raw almonds
- 1 Cup of raw cashews
- ½ Cup of dried sour cherries
- 2 Tablespoons of flax seeds
- ¼ Cup of chia seeds
- ½ Cup of black sesame seeds
- ½ Cup of unsweetened flaked coconut

Directions:

1. Prepare a baking sheet by lining it with a parchment paper
2. Preheat your oven to about 250° F
3. Add the coconut nectar, the olive oil, a sprig of about 4 inch of rosemary
4. In a medium bowl; add the coconut nectar, the olive oil, and vanilla, about 4 inch sprig of rosemary, 1 pinch of salt, a little bit of cayenne, and a little bit of black pepper.
5. Let your ingredients boil over a low heat; then chop the almonds and the cashews
6. Chop the cherries and mince about 8 needles of rosemary
7. Mix the almonds, the cashew, the cherries, the rosemary, the flax seeds, the chia seeds, the sesame seeds and the coconuts
8. Remove the sprig of rosemary from the heat
9. Pour the liquid over the top and stir
10. Adjust the seasoning; then spread your granola over the baking sheet
11. Bake the granola for about 40 minutes
12. Serve and enjoy!

Nutritional information

- Calories per serving – 158 calories
- Fat per serving –8.9 grams
- Saturated Fat – 1.2 gram
- Total Carbs per serving –13.9 grams
- Protein per serving – 8.1 grams

CHAPTER 6

DESSERT RECIPES

BAKED APPLES WITH CINNAMON

- ***Cooking Time: 30 minutes***
- ***Preparation Time: 5 minutes***
- ***Servings: 4***

- **NOTE:**

A QUICK AND very easy to make baked ad stuffed baked apples, this recipe is packed with flavors and with nutrients. Raisins and apples are rich in vitamins and when baked together, they provide the body with the energy it needs.

INGREDIENTS

- 5 apples
- 1 Cup of raisins
- ¼ Cup of walnuts
- ¼ Teaspoon of cinnamon
- ½ Teaspoon of natural vanilla extract
- ½ Cup of water

Directions:

1. Heat your oven to about 375° F; then core the apples and pierce it with the help of a fork
2. Mix the raisins, the nuts, cinnamon, and the vanilla in a bowl
3. Fill the center of the apples with the prepared mixture of the fruits
4. Put the stuffed apples into a glass baking tray; then cover the tray with an aluminum foil paper
5. Bake the apples for around 30 minutes in the oven
6. Serve and enjoy!

Nutritional information

- Calories per serving – 119.1 calories
- Fat per serving –4.2 grams
- Saturated Fat – 1.4 gram
- Total Carbs per serving –22.01 grams
- Protein per serving – 0.5 grams

PEACH BITES

- ***Cooking Time: 25 minutes***
- ***Preparation Time: 10 minutes***
- ***Servings: 6***

- **NOTE:**

Peaches are fruits that originate from Northwest China; this fruit has always been cherished for its various benefits. So, what can be better than making a delicious dessert made of peaches?

INGREDIENTS:

- 1 Cup of dried peaches
- 1 Cup of roasted almonds
- ½ Cup of shredded unsweetened coconut
- 1 Tablespoon of olive oil
- 1 Large egg

Directions:

1. Put the peaches, the almonds and the coconut into a food processor and pulse it
2. Drizzle in the olive oil and pulse for a few more seconds
3. In a large mixing bowl, combine the mixture with the egg and whisk very well
4. Make about 10 patties by rolling it; then press the dough and arrange the patties over a baking sheet
5. Bake your patties in the oven at a temperature of about 350°F for about 25 minutes
6. Serve and enjoy your peach patties!

Nutritional information

- Calories per serving – 150 calories
- Fat per serving –2.2 grams
- Saturated Fat – 0.3 gram
- Total Carbs per serving –13.1 grams
- Protein per serving – 3.3 grams

ALMOND MEAL SESAME CRACKERS

- *Cooking Time: 20 minutes*
- *Preparation Time: 5 minutes*
- *Servings: 8*

- **NOTE:**

Sesame seeds are considered as one of the most beneficial ingredients that can help you feel full in a short time. People, who use sesame in their daily meals, remain healthy as sesame is packed with nutrients.

INGREDIENTS:

- ½ Cup of almond meal
- 1/3 Cup of sesame seeds
- 1 Teaspoon of olive oil
- 1 Large egg white
- 1 Pinch of salt
- 1 Pinch of pepper

Directions:

1. Preheat your oven to about 365° F.
2. Put all the ingredients into a large bowl and mix very well
3. Put the mixture over a baking sheet; then cover it with another baking sheet
4. Roll the mixture with a rolling pin
5. Score the pastry with the back of your knife into pieces shaped into squares
6. Remove the baking paper from the top of your pastry and transfer it to a baking pan
7. Put the pastry in the oven for about 18 minutes
8. Serve and enjoy!

Nutritional information

- Calories per serving – 196 calories
- Fat per serving – 16 grams
- Saturated Fat – 2.01 gram
- Total Carbs per serving – 6 grams
- Protein per serving – 7.9 grams

ALMOND FLOUR MUFFINS

- ***Cooking Time: 20 minutes***
- ***Preparation Time: 5 minutes***
- ***Servings: 8***

- **NOTE:**

Paleo people have found that using Almond flour is a perfect choice as it is gluten-free. Almond flour is also excellent for its role in maintaining a healthy level of cholesterol and helps in maintaining a healthy heart. Besides, this dessert recipe is easy to make and packed with benefits

INGREDIENTS:

- 2 Cups of almond flour
- 2 Teaspoons of baking powder
- ¼ Teaspoon of salt
- ½ Cup of melted almond butter
- 4 Large eggs
- 1/3 Cup of water

- 1/3 Cup of maple syrup

Directions:

1. Preheat your oven to about 350° F.
2. Grease a baking 12 muffin-tins pan with cooking spray or butter
3. Mix the dry ingredients very well
4. Add the wet ingredients and mix very well
5. Pour your batter into the muffin tins.
6. Bake your muffins in the oven for about 25 minutes
7. Remove from the oven; then set the muffins aside to cool for about 10 minutes
8. Serve and enjoy your muffins!

Nutritional information

- Calories per serving – 184 calories
- Fat per serving –12.3 grams
- Saturated Fat – 1.2 gram
- Total Carbs per serving –12.7 grams
- Protein per serving – 7.0 grams

STRAWBERRY AND KIWI SMOOTHIE

- *Cooking Time: 5 minutes*
- *Preparation Time: 5 minutes*
- *Servings: 2*

- **NOTE:**

The combination of strawberries with kiwi is a natural and healthy combination that can destroy any illness and protects the body from any outside risk. This strawberry and kiwi smoothie is also refreshing and extremely delicious, you will enjoy it cold!

INGREDIENTS

- 1 and ½ cups of frozen roughly chopped strawberries
- 1 and ½ cup of roughly chopped frozen kiwi
- 8 Leaves of fresh mint
- 2 Oz of rum
- 2 Cups of crushed ice

Directions:

1. Mix the frozen strawberries with about 4 mint leaves
2. Add 1 oz of rum; 1 cup of ice; then blend the ingredients until it becomes smooth into a blender.
3. Pour the strawberry smoothie into glasses
4. Repeat the same process with the kiwis; then pour the strawberry mixture on top
5. Garnish with the fresh strawberries and the mint leaves.
6. Refrigerate your smoothie cold

Nutritional information

- Calories per serving – 180.2 calories
- Fat per serving – 1.7 grams
- Saturated Fat – 0.2 gram
- Total Carbs per serving –44.1 grams
- Protein per serving – 2.1 grams

CHAPTER 7
CONCLUSION

Junk food and fast food are the main causes of many rising diseases like diabetes, obesity and many other diseases. Nutritionists and physicians focused their efforts on finding a healthy diet that can save our lives and improve our health. And on this framework, Paleo diet was proved to be one of the most effective diets ever. Indeed, the popularity of the Paleo diet has spread all over the globe and it has become the favorite diet of Athletes. The Paleo diet has proven its success, especially in losing weight and the results were surprising to many people who managed to lose extra pounds in a very short period of time. While you might think that there is no existence for a perfect diet, the Paleo diet remains the best approach that can help us optimise our performance through what we eat and what we drink. You might have heard a lot about the Paleo diet, but the recipes that you will find in our book will allow you to taste the most delicious and healthiest recipes ever. Remember, this book complements our first Paleo book, and if you need more information and clarifications about the benefits of adopting the Paleo diet, then we encourage you to read our book ***"Paleo Diet cookbook for beginners"*** You can adapt all of the information you will find to your own needs and to your preferences.

THANKS FOR READING OUR BOOK

We are happy to grant you this book and we wish that
you have benefited from reading it. If you found
the Paleo recipes we have offered you delicious
and helpful; share it with the rest of your friends.
We value your reviews, and we are open to hear
from you. You can help others find our books by
leaving a review. All your feedbacks will
encourage us to keep writing delicious and
healthy recipe books that will help you lose
weight.
You won't regret reading our recipe books, and don't
forget to keep following our scrumptious recipes
for a longer and healthier life!